Patient and Family Education in Managed Care and Beyond

William Baragar (Barry) Bateman is a medical educator who is widely known for his expertise in primary care for diverse indigent populations, and for health promotion through lifestyle change. A Clinical Associate Professor of Medicine at the New York University School of Medicine, he served as Chief of Medicine and, until January 1999, as Medical Director of the Gouverneur Diagnostic and Treatment Center, an ambulatory care facility affiliated with NYU.

A graduate of the University of Michigan College of Medicine, Dr. Bateman is currently the Director of Business Development for the South Manhattan Healthcare Network, a vertically integrated health care system, including Gouverneur, Bellevue Hospital Center and Cohen-Goldwater Memorial Hospital, operated by the New York City Health and Hospitals Corporation. He maintains a clinical practice and continues to pursue his interest in clinical nutrition and preventive medicine.

Elizabeth J. Kramer is a Research Scientist in the Department of Medicine at New York University School of Medicine, and a medical writer. Her research and writing interests include patient and provider education; access to health care services, especially by the poor and underserved; women's health; immigrant health, and the delivery of culturally competent care to immigrant patients. She has been actively involved in patient education and writing about patient education at NYUMC's Cooperative Care Center. Her current activities include research on Type 2 diabetes in Chinese and Spanish-speaking immigrants, the development of educational materials for immigrant patients, and managed care education for health care providers. She is an alumna of New York University College of Arts and Sciences and the Johns Hopkins University School of Hygiene and Public Health. She is the editor of *Immigrant Women's Health: Problems and Solutions*, which was published by Jossey-Bass in 1999.

Kimberly S. Glassman is Director of the Case Management and Clinical Pathways Program at NYU Medical Center and former Director of Nursing of the Cooperative Care Center at the same institution. She has consulted and published internationally on involving patients and their families in their care and is an active speaker and writer on case management programs and the use of clinical pathways and guidelines to improve care. She is a graduate of the Massachusetts General Hospital School of Nursing, Hunter-Bellevue School of Nursing of the City University of New York, and New York University.

Patient and Family Education in Managed Care and Beyond

Seizing the Teachable Moment

William B. Bateman, *MD*
Elizabeth J. Kramer, *MPH*
Kimberly S. Glassman, *RN, MS*
Editors

 Springer Publishing Company

Springer Publishing Company, Inc.
536 Broadway
New York, NY 10012-3955

Acquisitions Editor: Ruth Chasek
Production Editor: Janice Stangel
Cover design by James Scotto-Lavino

99 00 01 02 03 / 5 4 3 2 1

Library of Congress Cataloging-in-Publication Data

Patient and family education in managed care : seizing the teachable
    moment / William B. Bateman, Elizabeth J. Kramer, and
    Kimberly S. Glassman, editors.
        p.   cm.
    Includes bibliographical references and index.
    ISBN 0-8261-1295-1 (hardcover)
    1. Patient education.   2. Managed care plans (Medical care)
I. Bateman, William B. (William Baragar)   II. Kramer, Elizabeth Jane.
    [DNLM: 1. Managed Care Programs—organization & administra-
tion—United States.   2. Health Services Needs and Demands—
United States.   3. Nurse-Patient Relations–United States.
4. Patient Education—methods—United States.   5. Physician-Patient
Relations—United States.   W 130 AA1 P25 2000]
R727.4.P372   2000
615.5'071—dc21
DNLM/DLC   99-37810
for Library of Congress   CIP

Printed in the United States of America

To Jo Ivey Boufford and Robert Massid, who inspired me to keep the patient first while thinking about the broader health system.

WBB

To Anthony J. Grieco, whose vision of patient and family education inspired us.

EJK and KSG

Contents

Part II: Working with Specific Patient Populations

Part III. Looking Ahead

Tables and Figures

Contributors

Steve Albert, M.P.H.
Director of HIV Services
Callen-Lorde Community Health
  Center
New York, New York

Wendy Berkowitz, M.D.
Clinical Instructor of Pediatrics
New York University School of
  Medicine
New York, New York

Julia A. Bucher, RN, Ph.D.
Associate Professor of Commu-
  nity Health Nursing
Bloomsburg University
Bloomsburg, Pennsylvania

Regina Butler, R.N.
Clinical Manager
Division of Hematology
Children's Hospital of
  Philadelphia
Philadelphia, Pennsylvania

Cara Cassino, M.D.
Assistant Professor of Medicine
New York University School of
  Medicine
Medical Director, Bellevue Hospi-
  tal Chest Clinic
New York, New York

Esther Chachkes, D.S.W.
Director of Social Work and Ther-
  apeutic Recreation
NYU Hospitals Center
New York, New York

**James E. Conlon, Jr., F.S.A.,
M.A.A.A.**
Consulting Actuary
Milliman and Robertson, Inc.
Albany, New York

Terry C. Davis, Ph.D.
Professor of Medicine and
  Pediatrics
Louisiana State University Medi-
  cal Center—Shreveport
Shreveport, Louisiana

Shelby L. Dietrich, M.D.
Associate Clinical Professor of
Pediatrics and Orthopedics
University of Southern California
    School of Medicine
(Retired) Director, Hemophilia
    Center
Huntington Hospital
Pasedena, California

Craig Epsom-Nelms, M.Ed.
former HIV Counselor Hemo-
    philia Treatment Center
North Carolina

Adeboye Francis, M.D.
Resident, Internal Medicine
The Brooklyn Hospital
Brooklyn, New York

S. Jody Heymann, M.D., Ph.D.
Director of Policy
Harvard University Center for
    Society and Health
Assistant Professor of Health and
    Social Behavior
Harvard School of Public Health
Boston, Massachusetts

Elizabeth Joglar, C.S.W.
HIV Case Management
    Consultant
New York City Health and
    Hospitals Corporation
New York, New York

Christine Kerr
Research Assistant
Harvard School of Public Health
Boston, Massachusetts

Jay Laudato, C.S.W.
Asssociate Executive Director
Callen-Lorde Community Health
    Center
New York, New York

Ruth Parker, M.D.
Associate Professor of Medicine
Emory University School of
    Medicine
Atlanta, Georgia

Joan Reibman, M.D.
Associate Professor of Medicine
New York University School of
    Medicine
Medical Director, Bellevue Hospi-
    tal Primary Care Asthma Clinic
New York, New York

**Susan Resnik, Dr. P.H.,
    C.H.E.S.**
Health Care Consultant
Facilitator, U.C.S.D. Medical
    School
DelMar, California

Eugenia L. Siegler, M.D.
Associate Professor of Clinical
    Medicine
New York University School of
    Medicine
Chief, Geriatrics
The Brooklyn Hospital
Brooklyn, New York

Selina Siu, M.D.
Attending Physician
Gouverneur Diagnostic and
    Treatment Center
New York, New York

Rona Vail, M.D.
Medical Director
Callen-Lorde Community Health
    Center
Clinical Assistant Professor of
    Medicine
New York University School of
    Medicine
New York, New York

Daniel R. Tobin, M.D.
Hospice Palliative Care
    Consultant
VA Network Upstate, New York
Director, the Life Institute for
    FairCare Education
Albany, New York

Mark V. Williams, M.D.
Associate Professor of Medicine
Emory University School of
    Medicine
Atlanta, Georgia

Foreword

Educating patients and their family members about their health may seem simple. Simple, at least until health care professionals attempt it. Providing patients and their family members with the relevant and timely information, skills, and support to fully participate in their care is an enormous undertaking that requires initial and sustained resources. This book provides a rich source of numerous very practical suggestions for patient and family education. The authors most skillfully identify the relevant issues in today's health care environment. Inclusion of Bringewatt's "triocular approach" to integrated care with chronic diseases, acute care, long-term care, and managed care is an especially helpful framework.

This much needed book brings together the challenges of patient and family education in the current health care environment of managed care. Active participation of patients and families in their care is essential for managed care to work well. Because HMOs are reimbursed on a fixed, capitated basis, there is an enormous potential to underserve and promote the underutilization of care. Therefore, not only do people need the prerequisite information, skills, and support to participate in their care, they also need knowledge about the health care services that are available in their managed care contracts and when to access them. The authors clearly identify the relevant issues in managed care organizations that affect individuals active participation or self-care.

Limited access to some services, and potential under service or reduced quality because of over subscription, gatekeeping and utilization controls, and delayed specialty referrals are all issues that directly affect active participation of patients and their families in HMOs.

This exciting new book is an easy read on the most current state-of-the-art and science of patient and family education. The authors artfully take the reader over some familiar and new ground. There are gentle reminders, for instance, of what collaborative care is, so the reader can re-learn this concept. There is an informative chapter on case management. The "new ground" content includes critical information regarding patients with limited health literacy, multiculturalism of patients and providers, and some creative features of existing programs.

This book is a must read for health care professionals who are struggling with how to provide quality patient and family education in a managed care environment.

Marylin J. Dodd
Professor and Associate Dean for Academic Personnel
School of Nursing, University of California, San Francisco

Foreword

Over the years, medical education has neglected patient education (not to mention family education) as a part of physician training. A survey of medical school curricula reveals that very little time is explicitly set aside for preparing graduates to become patient and family educators (Varner, 1998). This aspect of medical practice has been relegated to others—nurses, physician's assistants, and health educators. It is ironic that academic physicians, who thrive on teaching, have not provided leadership to this endeavor, and that managed care, which constrains the physicians' time, becomes the stimulus for considering it. However, it is not only managed care that provokes an interest in this topic, but also the new concern in medical education for medicine as a "population science," not merely a science for the individual patient. To the degree that managed care promotes attention to issues beyond the individual patient by directing concern to preventive and cost-effective interventions for defined populations (such as a group of enrollees), it may play a role in promoting patient and family education. In fact many believe that managed care has driven the disease management movement, which clearly was an inspiration for this book. It is worth pointing out, however, that the best disease management efforts have arisen in non-profit, staff-model managed care organizations, which preceded the recent wave of for-profit managed care companies (Bodenheimer, 1999).

Do managed care and medicine mix? Not very well, according to academic physicians and medical students who recently were interviewed (Simon, et al, 1999). In this survey, managed care fared worse than fee-for-service medicine in terms of continuity of care, quality of the doctor-patient-relationship, care for patients with chronic illness, care at the end of life, and minimizing ethical conflicts, i.e., in *personal health services*. Managed care outranked fee-for-service medicine only in providing preventive services, the avoidance of unnecessary care, the coordination of care and cost effectiveness, i.e., the *population health* aspects of health care delivery. Although the question, "How does managed care impact on your ability to provide patient and family education?" was not asked, I dare say the answer most likely would have been negative, since a majority of faculty complain of decreased time for teaching. It therefore is both remarkable and important that this book points to the opportunities for patient and family education afforded by managed care.

Perhaps managed care, which may be here in one form today and completely changed into another form tomorrow, is not the real enabler. Rather it is the growing emphasis in medical training on the dialectic between the individual and society. We should not be disturbed that a good medical education, like a good liberal arts education, does not prepare students to help corporate managed care clear its bottom line. But we should really be upset that medical education does not train our graduates to be superior patient and family educators. The value of this book is not in its association with managed care, but rather in its advocacy for and practical suggestions about extending the impact of the physician-patient encounter beyond the examining room or the bedside visit into the patient's life at home and in the community. It is about the physician's role as a teacher and how that can be maximized in collaboration with colleagues (nurses, social workers, health educators) by seizing the teachable moment in the encounter and extending it beyond the encounter through the use of multiple innovations, from the media and the "web" to community-based resources. And it is about the physician's role in shared decision-making with patients and with colleagues.

Further, it is not necessary to limit the physician's role as patient and family educator to topics that are confined to the patient's illness or preventable health risks. Should physicians provide information about their financial arrangements with a managed care company? I think so. We are aware that managed care companies are less enthusiastic about this kind of patient education, and some still include gag clauses which actually proscribe information sharing of this nature. Although historically they have been extremely conservative in their opinions about health system change, it is remarkable that 57% of the respondents to the survey mentioned above favored a single-payer national health system. In fact, what if physicians were to communicate their preferences about health system change to their patients and the public at large?

One premise of this book is that the old order in which the doctor was the unquestioned authority has been challenged by the growth of the power of the purchaser, and that this in turn, has led to a new emphasis on the importance of the patient, as consumer. However, purchaser and patient are not always one and the same. Corporate purchasers frequently focus on the bottom line, reducing patients' options. Nonetheless, there is no doubt that patients and their families, independent of the purchasers, are demanding more information and greater participation in medical decision making. This book helps all providers—physicians, nurses, social workers, health educators to seize the teachable moment by using creative tools and techniques to provide the most advanced patient and family education and guide patients and their families in their self-directed learning.

Oliver Fein
Associate Dean
Weill College of Medicine
Cornell University

Prologue

In the 1970s, many of us thought that health care was not subject to market forces because control of consumption came from the industry itself, not from the consumer. At the time, many assumed that meant market forces could not influence medical care. Now we realize our notion was as preposterous as believing that gravity will not influence us because we are flying in an airplane.

In the health care consumer revolution following the most recent attempt to establish a national health system, managed care oriented insurance companies gained the purchasing power of government, industry, and labor. This has been accomplished through the low premiums associated with managed care health insurance, and promises of better quality service. As this book is being written, managed care continues its rapid advancement to a dominant position in determining how health care is delivered in the United States.

Nonetheless, despite capturing and reshaping our health care delivery system, managed care is, at best, controversial among the professionals and institutions delivering health services. It also is increasingly the target of a rapidly emerging legislative backlash to prevent market forces from limiting access and costs of certain services. The fiscal incentives and "gatekeeper" role which physicians often assume in managed care has undermined the provider-patient relationship, and cast health care providers into adversarial roles with insurance companies as well as— sometimes—with their patients. Whether this eventually will result in blunting the impact of managed care, a return to fee-for-service, or the emergence of a new model such as integrated patient care, is still a matter of speculation.

Consistent in all of this is that physicians, nurses, and other health care professionals are still expected to treat patients. Further, as always, they will be judged by their patients on the basis of this relationship.

The need for effective partnerships between patients and their providers and among patients, their families, and providers has never been greater. Today, many procedures that were performed only on inpatients are now routinely done in the outpatient setting. Patients who are hospitalized are being discharged "quicker and sicker," and high technology care is being delivered more and more frequently in the home. Although it has been conclusively demonstrated that more can be done with less, the question of how much less and how much more remains.

As if this weren't enough change for health care providers, self-care is becoming more and more the mode, use of non-allopathic modalities is becoming more prevalent and, with the information explosion, nearly everyone has access to more information, all looking authoritative to consumers, but of highly variable quality. Nonetheless, patients and their families need us as advocates and educators. More than ever, our partnership with them is fundamental to the delivery of high quality preventive services and medical care.

This book is based on the premise that it is important for health care professionals who deliver services to have a dominant influence on health care, and that this influence is now threatened. The book begins with a recent history of our national search for a better way to obtain health care services. To meet the demands for efficacy and efficiency, the developing service delivery models rely heavily on patient and family self-care, as well as focused interdisciplinary teams, guided by carefully developed patient management tools.

This system does not leave room for the model primary care provider of 1970s television, Marcus Welby, M.D. Kind, caring, and skilled as he was, Dr. Welby would be too slow and too limited. Health care providers for the coming millennium need very different knowledge, skills, and attitudes. However, we still need the same trusted and caring relationships with our patients. We believe that this will come through using the tools of today's health care environment and seizing the moment to promote and guide our patients' health education.

This book is our attempt to assist health care providers in doing this; We hope we have been successful. The chapters that follow provide a background on how we got to where we are, the essentials of case management and clinical pathways development, strategies and resources for seizing the teachable moment, and dealing with individuals with special communication needs. They are followed by a series of chapters on clinical topics, including health promotion and disease prevention, the frail elderly, asthma, AIDS, hemophilia, and death and dying that illustrate both the importance of patient teaching as well as techniques for teaching required material. The final chapters deals with the interrelationships of providers and patients.

William B. Bateman
Elizabeth J. Kramer
Kimberly S. Glassman

Acknowledgments

This book could not have been written without a great deal of assistance from others. By lending their specific expertise, our contributors taught us as they helped to make this a unique book; their hard work is greatly appreciated. A number of individuals reviewed all or parts of the manuscript, and provided many suggestions for improving the final version. They include: Harrison G.Bloom, Anthony J. Grieco, Leonard Katz, Robert Like, Catharine Mintzer, and Liza Severance-Lossin. Technical assistance and research support were provided by James Beattie and Dorice Vieira of the Ehrman Medicaal Library at NYU, and by our assistants, Noris Douglas, Lydia Rodriguez and Mary Jane Ruppert. Special thanks are due to Ruth Chasek, Barbara Trocco, Bill Tucker, and everyone at Springer Publishing for their excellent editorial advice and prodigious work to expedite the production of the book. Finally, we thank our families for enduring our long hours, especially the many week-ends we worked, and sometimes sore spirits as we labored to deliver this book.

PART I
Concepts, Issues, and Strategies

Chapter 1

Managed Care: An Evolving Concept

William B. Bateman

Increasingly, our health care system is being shaped by managed care, but managed medical care no longer is what it was, and it is not expected to remain what it is (Ginzberg & Ostow, 1997; Kuttner, 1998). What has been constant since managed care began in 1929 is that its growth is directed by the purchasers of health care; it is not liked by organized medicine; it is based on prepayment for medical care, forcing providers to deliver services within a predetermined budget; and its impact on our health care system is steadily increasing.

Regardless of how they are organized, individual health services depend on effective relationships and communication between those who deliver care and patients, their families, or significant others. However, while the patient-provider relationship remains the *sine qua non* of effective medical care, the radical difference between the fee-for-service environment and that of managed care requires that health care providers adapt and develop new approaches to this relationship. Whether we like it or not, those who pay for health care are demanding easier and more friendly access to services at the price they are willing to pay. They also expect services to focus on health promotion and disease prevention, to be well-coordinated, and to be of high quality.

In this chapter we will outline the direction and nature of this dynamic and threatening service environment by taking a selective look at the history, accomplishments, and impact of managed care. The intent is to provide a picture of how better quality health care is being pursued and defined. From this, we can gain insights into the new approaches we must adopt or develop to take advantage of the opportunities, and avoid the dangers, as our health care system and managed care itself continue to evolve.

What Managed Care Is When It's Not Managed Cost

The strength of managed care's appeal to those who pay for health care is seen in its origins and achievements. The model was introduced in the United States in 1929 when people in Elk City, Oklahoma established a rural, farmers' cooperative health plan. A local physician organized leading farmers to sell shares to raise money for a new hospital. Shareholders, in turn, received medical care at a discounted rate with payment of annual dues. Five years later, that plan had 600 member families, and the founding physician had added four new specialists and a dentist to the roster of service providers available to plan members. In 1934, a prepaid, comprehensive health service plan, in which two physicians agreed to provide comprehensive services for 2,000 water company employees at a predetermined rate was born in Los Angeles (MacColl, 1966). Although these and other early managed care plans encountered opposition from medical societies, managed care continued to expand, as more and more organized purchasers of health services found it to be a means of getting better access to the health services they wanted at the price they could afford.

Despite the many dramatic and unprecedented advances in the effectiveness of health care that took place between 1930 and 1960, such as the development of antibiotics and the discovery of insulin, a portion of the health care market sought better value, pursuing both a different understanding of high-quality service and a lower price. Thus over the next three decades, more plans were shaped by a belief that higher-quality services could be provided at a lower price than was available under fee-for-service.

This formative period in managed care launched what Robert Kuttner has aptly dubbed the "socially oriented forms of managed care" (Kuttner, 1998, p. 1558). The value and durability of the "socially oriented" model is appreciated by reflecting on the accomplishments and age of some of the prominent members of this group: Kaiser Permanente founded in 1942; the Group Health Cooperative of Puget Sound, and the Health Insurance Plan of Greater New York, both founded in 1947; and the Group Health Plan of Minneapolis, founded in 1957.

"Socially oriented" plans emphasize prevention, patient education, and cost-effective care. They also provide feedback to providers to generate "best practices" by improving and monitoring the processes and outcomes of patient care. This emphasis has provided many advances in the delivery of health services, and with the parallel movement to expand attention to primary care, it can be credited with greatly expanding the field of health services research itself.

Health Services Research and Managed Care

A review of some key concerns in health services research that are specifically addressed by the managed care model provides a strong image of what is driving the purchasers of health care toward managed care. It also gives providers clear direction to improve care and attract the payers.

A basic concern of managed care is the desire to improve cost-efficiency. The belief that care under fee-for-service will be inefficient is fundamental to the premise that something is wrong with fee-for-service practice, because fee-for-service care offers no financial incentive to reduce waste and, in fact, rewards it. An abundance of data supports this theory. Research shows inexplicable variations in clinical practices, and in international comparisons of health expenditures and outcomes.

In 1973, John Wennberg and Alan Gittelsohn reported wide and clinically indefensible variations in medical practice. For example, the rates of surgery in given localities were more dependent on the number of surgeons than on population or disease characteristics (Wennberg & Gittelsohn, 1973). It rapidly became accepted that care decisions often were made poorly, and that more services were being used than necessary. With waste and inefficiency apparent in medical practice, opinion spread that our health system under fee-for-service was inefficient.

A recently published study compared the "health-care efficiency" in the United States with nine other developed countries (Kjellstrand, Kovithavongs, & Szabo, 1998). The study derived a "health-care efficiency index" by multiplying the mean per capita health expenditure by the mean death rate for six "avoidable" causes of mortality (tuberculosis, cervical cancer, chronic rheumatic heart disease, hypertensive disease, cerebrovascular disease, and appendicitis), and dividing it by the individual country's per capita expenditure times the death rates for the same diseases. The United States was ranked least efficient among the 10, with an efficiency index that was nearly 1/3 that of Australia, which was rated the most efficient of the ten countries.

The index related expense and health outcome on an equal basis; therefore, countries were ranked as highly efficient in very contrasting ways. New Zealand was second "most efficient" due to spending so little that this offset the worst overall outcomes among the compared countries. In contrast, Canada, which was rated third most efficient, had the best outcomes while spending a great deal. Thus, while one can debate the merits of being ranked high in "health care efficiency," this and an abundance of other data identifying the United States as spending large sums but getting relatively little in return generates much of the search for a better approach to delivering care. Whether managed care will provide this better approach still is not known, but it does align the incentive of providers with the desire of purchasers to control costs.

Fueled by a belief that patients can get more from a system that has financial incentives to improve health, cost control in managed care is approached by increasing the focus on health promotion and disease prevention, as well as by providing interdisciplinary support to prevent waste and, in better developed systems, to facilitate optimal care. In the service environment, this translates into:

- Offering an array of health promotion services and using health promotion in marketing managed care organizations (MCOs);
- Utilization review and management;
- Collaborative care (care, case, and disease management); and
- Quality assurance and improvement

MCOs and Health

Many MCOs promote themselves by telling potential buyers about their programs and accomplishments in health promotion and disease prevention. This is done both by proudly displaying their attention to immunizations and early disease detection (i.e., screening), and sometimes by offering discounted access to membership in exercise facilities or for the purchase of exercise equipment. Patient education materials on nutrition and fitness also are provided to plan members through newsletters, pamphlets, and the Internet. If direct service providers encourage and help their patients to use this material, we are both taking advantage of tools that can improve the health of our patients, and showing interest and ability in something for which our patients are looking in health care. If we do not do this, we are sending a very negative message: that we are less interested in promoting health than a health insurance company.

An additional approach used by some MCOs to advance an image of aggressively promoting health is to offer an array of services that are far from the mainstream of American medicine, but increasingly popular with health-conscious people. While many of us still bristle at the potential dangers and often, little scientific support for such approaches as vitamin and mineral supplements, herbals, acupuncture, therapeutic touch, massage, homeopathy, traditional Chinese medicine, and even chiropractic, our patients' belief in and use of these services is increasing dramatically (Eisenberg et al., 1998). Knowledge about these alternative therapies and their scientific foundations, or lack thereof, also is expanding (Fontanarosa & Lundberg, 1998). Again, if we know whether our patients are using or should be using any of these approaches, we are both promoting their health and showing interest in and knowledge about services they seek. Failure to show interest in this particular sphere of health-seeking behavior shows more than a parochial attitude; it can have serious sequelae.

Utilization Review and Management

Utilization review and management (UR) has emerged out of the desire to reduce unjustified variations in practice. Although it is one of the most despised and potentially damaging components of managed care, and has produced a number of problems, UR has had some positive results.

At its roots, UR is simply a way of executing "evidence-based" medicine. It is what is used as "evidence," and what happens when care plans do not fit the "evidence-based" criteria, that determine a good or a bad experience for patient, provider, or both. The dominant, contrasting approaches used are, on the one hand, applying practice norms as the evidence to define criteria for appropriate care and, on the other hand, using expert opinion and study data to define appropriateness criteria.

The normative approach uses averages, e.g., average lengths of stay, to define the line between acceptable and unacceptable. The problem with this approach is the assumption that an individual's care should fit within the average, potentially ignoring that there are reasons for practices, like data, to distribute all cases along a bell-shaped curve.

The expert or study-driven approach uses expert opinion and research evidence to determine the appropriateness of care by looking at factors that define patient needs based on specific characteristics of individuals, not just the group in which their diagnosis places them. While this seems to be the most thoughtful and valid approach, this model is still limited by the many areas that lack sufficient evidence to really make a research, evidence-based decision that actually fits the patient whose care is in question. The wide variations in expert opinion and the biases that influence opinion, even if expert, also are limiting factors.

Both approaches are used, and both can positively influence the quality of care, and not just contain the costs. In any case, if we health care providers better understand where utilization criteria come from and how they are used, we can better help our patients understand when the MCO is helping us provide better care, and when it is getting in the way. This also will help us better influence UR itself.

Collaborative Care (Care, Case, and Disease Management)

The real trouble comes not so much from which approach is being used for UR, but rather what is done when the care plan does not meet the criteria for approval. UR that does not provide either support for or direction to an acceptable approach can be referred to as the "GOMER" or "Get Out of My Emergency Room" approach (House of God). When direction is added, it becomes a "best practices" approach and, with supports, a care-managed approach.

As long as care was fully reimbursed under fee-for-service, there was no fiscal incentive to support providers with interdisciplinary teams to facilitate more effective and efficient patient care. However, with "profit" coming from savings due to better health or more efficient service delivery, managed care rewards the creation of teams to support better outcomes and maximum efficiency. This orientation has led to programs for disease management, case management, and care management, which have developed rapidly with some dramatic successes. However, much more continues to be promised than is delivered (Curtiss, 1997).

A vision of how much care can be improved under care management can be readily imagined by reflecting on the following questions. When managing patients with many complex problems, or a chronic disease that requires a great deal of self-care, do you really believe that a doctor working alone can produce better results than can be achieved by a dedicated interdisciplinary team? It seems quite possible that the team can fail due to poor execution, but can we believe that they won't do better when they are functioning optimally?

Many believe that the answer to the above questions is that a dedicated interdisciplinary team will produce better results, possibly at a lower cost. As a result, "collaborative care models" (disease management, case management, and care management), are rapidly being developed for and by MCOs. In a 1997 survey, 94% of MCOs projected that they expected increased resources and influence from disease management programs (Curtiss, 1997).

Collaborative care also has been demonstrated to produce superior results in well-designed studies. For example, a randomized trial evaluating the efficacy of a "physician-directed, nurse-managed, home-based case-management system for coronary risk factor modification" in post-myocardial infarction patients was considerably more effective in achieving smoking cessation (17% greater than usual care, $p = 0.03$), reducing LDL cholesterol (107 mg/dL vs. 132 mg/dL, $p = 0.0001$), and increasing functional capacities (9.3 METS vs. 8.4 METS, $p = 0.001$) (Debusk et al., 1994).

The focus of collaborative care with which we are most familiar is discharge planning under the influence of Diagnosis Related Groups (DRG) payment; in essence, this is risk-adjusted, prepaid hospital care. In hospital care and discharge management, case management is the standard practice used by hospitals to decrease the length of stay. It has been enormously effective. The challenging opportunity now is moving this approach to the outpatient setting for chronic disease management, health promotion, and disease prevention.

The race is on to produce collaborative care services that improve health outcomes while controlling or reducing overall costs. In the "Health Project Consortium" Fries et al. (1998) are looking for the "moral high ground" of such services. They astutely define their goal as not only reducing the demand for health services (e.g., gatekeeper-type activities), but also the actual need for such services (i.e., producing better health). In their review of health education programs designed to decrease both health risks and costs, they found 32 effective programs. They also identified "multiple model [chronic disease management . . .] programs that have both improved health and substantially decreased costs" (Fries et al., 1998, p. 76).

While not all collaborative care programs will add value to the general practice environment, their great potential for benefiting patients while also reducing costs is clear. Health care providers who are aware of the programs to which their patients have access, those who work to improve care management, and those who help their eligible patients to participate will be in practices that benefit from these approaches. Those who do not will have to compete on their own.

Quality Assurance and Improvement

The goals of health care quality improvement mirror those of health care under managed care: to adhere to standards of quality, eliminate unjustifiable variations, and satisfy patients. The strong role of managed care in quality assessment in general is abundantly clear with the increasing use of the Health Plan Employer Data and Information Set (HEDIS) indicators to measure quality of health care on a national basis. HEDIS emerged in the early 1990s when organized managed care joined large employers (as major purchasers of health care) to define quality standards.

MCOs are now organized nationally to focus on quality and report it through the National Committee for Quality Assurance (NCQA), which has assumed the administration of HEDIS and the role of accreditor. However, although the goals are clear and admirable, their execution is still highly criticized. "Most quality monitoring in these . . . MCO . . . groups assesses overuse rather than underuse" (Kerr, Mittmasn, Hays, Leake, & Brook, 1996). And, the measures only scratch the surface of cost-effective, ethical medicine (Berwick, 1996; Blumenthal, 1996; Blumenthal, 1996; Blumenthal & Epstein, 1996; Brook, 1996; Chassin, 1996).

However, managed care does add new dimensions to the promotion of quality care. For example, the American Association of Health Plans has organized an Immunization Task Force with NCQA, the Pharmaceutical Manufacturers Association, the American College of Physicians, the

American Academy of Pediatrics, the American Academy of Family Physicians, the National Vaccine Advisory Committee, Immunization Action Coalition, and the Centers for Disease Control and Prevention in an ex-officio status. Their mission is "to identify and discuss a collective needs assessment for MCOs necessary to meet the immunization challenge and protect the health and long-term well-being of our population" (p. 3). Under fee-for-service care a health promotion initiative like this was only a concern for public health. With managed care, the health of the enrolled population is the concern of the health insurance company whether or not individuals come in for services (Immunization Task Force, 1998).

The impact of managed care's focus on pursuing and reporting quality care for populations is even more apparent in its influence on the nation's largest insurer, Medicaid. Since its inception in 1965, Medicaid has grown to pay for the health services of roughly 41.3 million Americans with low incomes who are elderly, disabled, blind, receiving public assistance, or among the working poor. In 1997, Medicaid expended $159.9 billion, or 12.4% of our total health payments. Every state but Alaska now uses some form of managed care in its Medicaid program (Iglehart, 1999). While this shift to managed care was heavily motivated by a desire to contain costs, for many states it also has stimulated the first comprehensive assessment of the quality of services provided to Medicaid recipients (Landon, Tobias, & Epstein, 1998). This has yielded some very positive results. For example, in the early 1990s, New York State began monitoring access to services and HEDIS measures of quality on an annual basis for Medicaid recipients who voluntarily enrolled in a Medicaid managed care program. This has resulted in greatly improved access to services, and ever-improving rates in health promotion and disease prevention indicators such as immunizations, mammography, and retinal examinations for people with diabetes mellitus.

Nonetheless, the still unanswered question is: What is the evidence that managed care, as opposed to fee for service, offers a superior approach to health care? While the findings show much that is wrong with the execution of managed care, not surprisingly, some assessments of health care under managed care have shown favorable outcomes for patients in managed care compared with those who received fee-for-service care.

For example, one study assessed the process and outcomes of the care of more than 2000 patients with unstable angina who were treated in multiple settings. Compared with fee-for-service, managed care patients were more likely to receive care from a cardiologist (74% vs. 69%), more likely to be triaged to intensive or coronary care units (46% vs. 37%), more likely to be treated with beta blockers during hospitalization (60% vs. 54%), and more likely to be discharged on aspirin and beta blockers. While in-hospital catherization rates were lower in the managed care group, in-hospital mortality was the same (Every et al., 1998). These findings prompted one observer to write: "One interpretation of this study is that managed care patients actually received superior care" (Lee, 1998, p. 2).

However, comparisons of managed care and fee-for-service care are difficult to interpret. For example, concerns that managed care seeks cheap care, not better care, can lead to criticisms of managed care, even when outcomes under managed care appear to be superior. For example, recognizing that the worst outcome in critical care can be extending the suffering prior to death, and not death itself, Cher and Lenert (1997) compared the use of "potentially ineffective care" (PIC) in 81,494 Medicare patients admitted to an intensive care unit. Nearly 5% (3914), of the patients experienced PIC and used 21.6% of the total intensive care unit resources. Those in managed care Medicare programs were 25% less likely than those in fee-for-service Medicare to have experienced PIC. However, the finding that patients in a managed care plan were more likely to be protected from "injudicious . . . and expensive . . . use of critical care near the end of life" (Curtis & Rubenfeld, 1997, p. 1026) was questioned on the basis of whether the findings were an artifact of the different billing incentives or of patient selection between managed care and fee-for-service. Also, the appropriateness of reducing the PIC was questioned, as the 100-day mortality in the managed care group was 8% higher and they experienced 9% more hospitalizations during the subsequent year (Curtis & Rubenfeld, 1997).

Further, when conditions that lack clear standards for the appropriateness of care are studied, we cannot even tell when better care is delivered. For example, Goldzweig et al. (1997) compared cataract extraction rates in prepaid and fee-for-service Medicare populations in California. The study included 43,387 staff-model HMO enrollees, 19,050 independent practice association enrollees, and 47,150 fee-for-service beneficiaries. After controlling for age, sex, and diabetes mellitus, the fee-for-service beneficiaries were twice as likely to have undergone a cataract extraction. However, given the lack of clear measures of appropriateness, we do not know if this represents overuse in the fee-for-service group, or underuse in the prepaid group.

The importance of assessing all important aspects of the question, as well as the difficulty of trying to control costs, is well illustrated by a study which shows that attempts to save in one area can lead to increased costs in others, and even fail to hold down the costs in the targeted area. The managed care outcomes project was a longitudinal prospective study to examine variations in clinical and resource use among HMO patients over a one-year period (Horn, 1996). Five diseases which require pharmaceutical-intensive treatment and outpatient management—otitis media, atraumatic joint pain or arthritis, epigastric pain or ulcers, hypertension, and asthma—were selected based on the following criteria: high prevalence, having a wide variation among patients in terms of disease severity, the number of office visits, and drug utilization. Except for otitis media, limitations on drug availability were associated not only with higher use of office visits, emergency services and hospital admissions, but with a higher drug cost and drug count as well.

In defining the quality of most products, the consumer perspective is a sort of gold standard. However, we have only begun to assess and understand consumer perspectives in health care. For example, data are accumulating which indicate that patients (like health care providers) view amenities such as cleanliness and food, that are prominent in patient satisfaction studies, as very different from quality of care. Studies also suggest that assessing "satisfaction" is inadequate, as patients can be satisfied with low-quality care and dissatisfied with high-quality care. Thus, when we report quality, or for that matter, even when we report patient satisfaction, it is still with a very limited understanding of what our patients really want. Accordingly, the federal Agency for Health Care Policy and Research supports the "Consumer Assessment of Health Plans" project that is sorely needed if we are ever to validly compare approaches to health care and inform ourselves as well as our patients about quality health care (Cleary & Edgman-Levitan, 1997).

However, while our patients undoubtedly want to know whether or not they are getting high-quality services, informing them has had mixed effects on the care they receive. For example Longo et al. (1997) assessed the impact of an obstetrics consumer report on hospital behavior and found that the quality of hospital services and clinical outcomes improved after the report (Longo, Land, & Schramm, 1997). On the other hand, when Schneider and Epstein (1996) assessed the impact of a *Consumer Guide to Coronary Artery Bypass Graft Surgery*, they found that although 82% of the cardiologists and all of the cardiac surgeons were aware of the guide, it had very little influence on their referral recommendations, and they felt it had introduced a barrier to care for severely ill patients (Schneider & Epstein, 1996).

Whether managed care does or does not improve health services, it is producing major challenges for the primary resources that advance professional skills and the effectiveness of medical care itself. The decrease in hospital use and dramatic reduction in lengths of stay is reducing both the budgets of hospitals and their usefulness in medical education. Further, the emphasis on decreased referrals is contrary to the practice habits in most academic medical centers. While both of these factors are increasing the importance of teaching and research in outpatient settings, the efficiencies required in the practices of primary care providers severely limit the time for teaching and decrease the amount of responsibility that trainees can assume as well (Culbertson, 1996; Iglehart, 1995). Carey and Engelhard (1996, p. 839) conclude, "The extent to which managed care will ultimately alter the traditional role of academic health centers in the American health care system is unclear, but successful adaptation in the short term will require them to respond broadly, flexibly, and in a timely fashion to the anticipated health care scene." The same can be said for the entire health care system.

It is positive to note that managed care organizations and academic health centers are entering into collaborative relationships to support advances in medical service and directly pursue their common goals within their discordant cultures (Donahue et al., 1996).

When Managed Care Becomes Managed Costs

Managed care is not being molded solely by the ideals reviewed in the beginning of this chapter. Profit motives of providers, insurance companies, and shareholders have become very strong, and the subject of intense debate. Many observers trace the origins of the "market-oriented form of managed care" (Kuttner, 1998) to passage of the federal HMO Act in 1973, which enabled managed care plans to expand with support from grants, contracts, and loans. This enabled an explosive and extensive expansion of this model of care. HMO membership increased by nearly 20 million between 1976 and 1986, and then expanded by another 40 million in the following decade. The dramatic increase from 1986 to 1996 was boosted by the failed Clinton Health Plan and the subsequent market-driven pursuit of health care reform in the form of greatly reduced costs and managed care. Membership expanded by 9 million from 1990 through 1993, and then exploded by 22 million from 1993 through 1996, as the market sought, and, at least temporarily, gained health insurance at substantially reduced costs (American Association of Health Plans). This dramatic growth is likely to decrease, as MCOs lose the ability to hold down costs substantially (Freudenheim, 1998). It will be interesting to see whether MCOs can go beyond the accusation that "managed care has, so far, served us as a different way to pay for medical care, not a better way to provide it" (Kilborn, 1998).

The good and the bad in the evolution of managed care can be viewed by comparing the industry's self-portrayal to its customers to that emphasized to its business partners. Most simply stated, the customers are sold a product which promises comprehensive services, a personal doctor, the choice of doctors, higher-quality care, and an emphasis on health promotion and disease prevention, all at a lower premium. However, the market-oriented plans offer a low "medical-loss ratio," meaning that to attract business partners and shareholders, they seek to pay as small a percentage of the health insurance premium as possible to the direct providers of health care services. To achieve this they add several cynical features to the "socially-oriented model" to put barriers between patients and the care they want, and arrange to pay less to the direct providers of care, if they pay at all. The results of this split personality provide a dramatically different picture of what managed care achieves.

In comparing the care of 402 stroke patients treated by an HMO with that of 408 fee-for-service patients, Retchin, Brown, Yeh, Chu, and Moreno (1997) found that the HMO patients were less likely to go to rehabilitation facilities, a standard of practice for stroke patients, and less likely to return home, a desired outcome. The editorial comment on this study asks the question: "Is this another example of the new medical environment in which older individuals will be deprived of appropriate care to increase corporate profits or to reward physicians who benefit financially from withholding care?" (Webster & Feinglass, 1997).

However, while a worthy concern, it is a gross oversimplification to depict the strong pressure from the profit motive as entirely negative. Among other things, the investment capital it makes available has accelerated physical plant improvements and advances in information technology. Market forces also have had a profound influence on the service-delivery model for managed care. In fact, managed care plans have moved from a staff model HMO to the same point-of-service delivery models offered under fee-for-service or indemnity plans. Indeed, the diversity that has emerged goes well beyond the classic four: staff, independent practice association (IPA), preferred provider organization (PPO), and network. Mixed-models now exist, and a "tremendous heterogeneity . . . of plan types" have emerged out of large integrated delivery systems, all with differing ways of influencing the quality of care under managed care (Landon, Wilson, & Cleary, 1998). Managed care is no longer what it was, and, at the level of patients accessing services, it is mimicking indemnity plans. However, as it does this to attract customers, it is increasingly experiencing problems in keeping the cost of services within the price the payer wants to pay. This tension between providing low-cost insurance and meeting the demands for services undoubtedly will continue to profoundly modify the healthcare environment. The question for direct providers of medical care may not be so much "Will managed care continue its rapid growth and dominate in the future?" as "What should I do to provide good services and make a living in this era?", where the cliché, "Change is the only constant in life," has special meaning.

Health Service Delivery in our Changing Environment

"When the pace of change outside an organization exceeds the pace of change inside it, the end (i.e., demise) is near."
John R. Walter, President of AT&T

"Physicians . . . and other health care providers . . . have a golden opportunity to regain a leadership role in health care by publicly advocating for and practicing quality of care assurance, especially when such measures pertain to steadfast care of vulnerable, high-cost, high-risk patients. We need to show by our actions that we do not consider health care to be just another private consumer good to be efficiently regulated by the marketplace" (Webster & Feinglass, 1997).

With our health care system changing rapidly, we too must change briskly. I believe that the system functions best when those who need services understand both health and the system, and gain that understanding from their healthcare providers. Currently, this is not the case. Alternatively, they receive information from advertisements, legislative initiatives, political agendas, insurance companies, and managers of employee benefit packages. We must adapt our practices to deliver the product the purchaser wants, and educate our patients to take full advantage of their health plans, as well as to understand other available options.

To get our patients' attention, we must continuously improve our ability to meet the key objectives they are pursuing. Our patients must know that we support their pursuit of lower costs, friendlier and easier access, a personal physician, the ability to choose physicians, high quality, and an ability to assess quality, a focus on health promotion and disease prevention, and comprehensive services. Patient education is one of the most important, if not the only, vehicle that can serve all of these often competing, consumer-generated objectives for health care. We must focus on it in everything we do.

Informed patients can lower costs by adopting healthy lifestyles, practicing good self-care, and using services only as needed. Access to our services becomes friendlier and easier when patients know how to gain all levels of access they need: telephone, emergency, immediate nonemergent, and by appointments. Primary care providers become more personal when patients know their names and some personal information about them. Patients feel that they have more freedom to choose and use specialists when they know the qualifications and performance record of particular providers and when they know why a particular consultation or test is or is not needed. Our patients can better understand what quality health care is if we tell them how it is measured and how well we do. They must be motivated and aware to benefit from health promotion and disease prevention. Knowledgeable patients can make more effective use of comprehensive services.

But how many of us are prepared to meet this ambitious agenda? How do we get the time? We must use all available resources and organize ourselves and our offices toward this end. We must become knowledgeable about supporting activities in our patients' insurance companies. We must make better use of technology and interdisciplinary teams in all health care settings. We must seize the moment and engage our patients and ourselves in the pursuit of better value in health care.

Chapter 2

Strategies for Patient Teaching: How to Seize the Teachable Moment

Elizabeth J. Kramer, Julia A. Bucher, Kimberly S. Glassman, and Selina Siu

One of the principal findings of the United States Preventive Services Task Force is that clinicians are more likely to help their patients prevent future disease by asking, educating, and counseling them about personal health behaviors than by performing physical examinations or tests. In other words, "Talking is more important than testing" (Woolf, Jonas, & Lawrence, 1995, p. xxxvii).

Today more than ever, individuals are responsible for their own health maintenance, for modifying their behavior to reduce the risks of various chronic diseases, and for managing multiple chronic illnesses with complex therapeutic regimens, some of which require technologically sophisticated equipment. Providers have less time to teach and counsel patients on a one-to-one basis. At the same time the consumer movement and microcomputers have helped many patients, particularly of the Baby Boom generation and younger, to become increasingly more sophisticated about health care and seek information about health problems. This chapter describes strategies and resources that will help health care professionals to seize teachable moments with patients and their families and, in the process, enable them to assume greater responsibility for their own health maintenance and disease management. It also will describe some of the ways in which patients acquire their own information, with a focus on Internet resources and news media.

Everyone Is a Teacher

Education is a team effort, and every health care professional and support person has an educational component to his or her role. The Worcester-Area Trial for Counseling in Hyperlipidemia (WATCH) demonstrated that a systematic approach to education that includes training of office practice support staff as well as physicians can improve patient outcomes (Ockene, Heebert, & Ockene, 1996).

In a program called MULTI-FIT, a systems approach in secondary prevention used nurse case managers to do multiple risk factor intervention in patients recovering from myocardial infarctions. Education and counseling, which included individualized interventions for smoking cessation, exercise training, and dietary treatment for dyslipidemia, was available for 1 year following discharge. Those who required lipid-lowering medications were treated according to protocol by the nurse case managers. A randomized controlled clinical trial was used to evaluate the program. At 1 year, significant differences were noted in functional capacity, biochemically confirmed smoking cessation, and plasma LDL-C values in the intervention group, compared to those who received usual care (Debusk et al., 1994).

A study of chronic disease management in heart failure patients demonstrated that coordinated multidisciplinary care can substantially decrease rehospitalization for heart failure (Rich, Beckham, & Wittenberg, 1995).

In addition to the traditional members of the professional team, such as physicians, nurses, and social workers, we believe that nursing assistants, peer educators, and most office personnel who are properly trained and supervised can also do some patient teaching.

A Few Caveats About Teaching and Learning

The Domains of Learning

There are three types of learning that patients and their families need to accomplish: cognitive, which expands the knowledge base; affective, which is important for changing attitudes; and psychomotor, for developing skills to perform physical tasks such as capillary blood glucose monitoring. It is important to identify the domain of learning as it influences the choice of method used for teaching. Cognitive function has an important bearing upon individuals' abilities to perceive and understand information that is conveyed to them.

In recent years there has been greater recognition of the importance of psychosocial and behavioral factors in health status. Attitudes can strongly influence people's willingness to learn, their beliefs in what is being conveyed, and their adherence to prescribed therapeutic regimens. Anxiety and apprehension also can strongly affect individuals' abilities to learn, as well as their physical status.

Psychomotor abilities are extremely important in this age of increasing technological complexity, where patients and their families frequently have to use home dialysis machines, maintain vascular access ports, and administer and monitor total parenteral nutrition. However, many more mundane activities, such as home monitoring of blood glucose, injecting insulin, and even properly inserting contact lenses and organizing medicines also require psychomotor skill.

Provider-Patient Communication

Patients and families need more than clinical expertise from their health care providers. They expect and are entitled to friendly, concerned, and empathetic professionals who are willing to take the time to answer their questions. The health care provider can encourage patient and family participation by presenting a collegial demeanor and encouraging an open dialogue. Patients and their families have worthy insights and contributions to make to their health care which can be facilitated by asking open-ended questions and responding to all of the questions they ask (Enslow & Adler, 1972).

Effective communication between patient and professional is the most essential aspect of the relationship because it improves the accuracy of a medical history and systems review, and increases patients' adherence to medical regimens (Becker & Maiman, 1975) and satisfaction with the care they receive (Greene et al., 1994). Miscommunication can lead to unnecessary anxiety, loss of confidence in the medical care system, and possible health problems due to misunderstanding of schedules, therapeutic regimens, or contraindications to medications (Phelan, Kramer, Grieco, & Glassman, 1996). Expectations of good provider-patient communication are summarized in Table 2.1. Effective communication between provider and patient lays the foundation for learning.

How We Learn

Children learn in structured and often directed environments. Adult learners, on the other hand, usually are self-directed. They need a sense of control over their environment to establish a level of comfort, and they are most likely to learn when they and their teachers establish goals and objectives together, especially in one-on-one counseling. Where much of the teaching occurs in group sessions and is protocol-driven (e.g., in diabetes education or preparation for open heart surgery), expectations of both the teacher and the learner should be clarified by stating the educational goals and objectives at the beginning of the session.

Table 2.1   Expectations of Good Provider-Patient Communication

1. Office or clinic staff who are calm and responsive to patients, and who value patients' need for appointments which are promptly and efficiently scheduled and on time.
2. Providers who maintain eye contact and speak to the patient with respect and at a level of medical complexity which he or she can understand.
3. Practitioners who use empowering language and limit their use of jargon.
4. Providers who take the time with patients to listen to their symptoms and concerns.
5. Providers who create an atmosphere that provides a level of comfort for patients to verbalize their questions about medical conditions and procedures and express their fears about the unknown.
6. Providers who have non-judgmental attitudes toward individuals who are different than they. This will allow patients to honestly discuss sensitive issues such as sexual orientation and behavior, drug and alcohol behavior, and illegal activities or behaviors which differ from community norms.
7. Providers who respect the concerns of all patients regardless of their race or age and will take all symptoms seriously rather than assigning easy labels such as "menopausal," "teenage behavior," "crock," or "so like that group."
8. Providers who explain the reasons for tests, when the results will be available, and how to get those results.
9. Providers who actively build partnerships which involve each patient in his/her health care, addressing barriers to behavior change, and working together to identify alternative solutions.
10. Providers who are available for follow-up questions and who return telephone calls in a timely manner.

Older learners bring a great deal of life experience to their educational encounters. This must be recognized and valued to make patient education meaningful. To learn rapidly, adults need to integrate new ideas with established ones. If the old and the new are in conflict, it takes a long time to change beliefs. Adults also take fewer risks when it comes to trying new solutions. In addition, they may have fears of the hospital and of diagnostic and therapeutic technology, and they may feel that they cannot succeed in rehabilitation settings. Depression can be a compounding problem which complicates learning. These issues make it extremely important to evaluate what has been learned.

The Educational Process

Overall, the education process has four components: assessment, planning, implementation, and evaluation.

Assessment

Patients' prior experience with the health care delivery system can be a barrier to acceptance of health messages and communication from the health care professional. The more the professional can learn about the patient's lifestyle, ethnicity, socioeconomic status, occupation, religion, language, family group or affiliation, values and beliefs, and knowledge of how and where a patient gets his or her health information, the more likely the success of the educational interventions.

Patient assessment also should include questions such as: Who besides the patient will be involved in his or her care? Will he or she be alone, and if so, will he or she be able to take care of him or herself? If not, are there family members available who can help? What about close friends, other health care professionals, personal care workers, nannies, school teachers, or supervisors at work? Teachers and work supervisors frequently need to know about and be prepared to render assistance to those with a number of medical problems, among them severe diabetes, seizure disorders, and bleeding problems.

Determination of the factors which may impede learning is an important part of the assessment. A number of physical conditions can make learning difficult including pain, manual dexterity problems, medication effects, and sensory impairments. Past experiences, beliefs and values, language, financial worries, availability of resources, and lack of an adequate support system are additional factors. Learning difficulties can be overcome by the use of appropriate media, a receptive and nonjudgmental attitude on the part of the educator, having adequate time, adapting to variations in learning styles, and paying attention to differing values and lifestyles. Enhancing patient motivation requires careful assessment of their desires and their reasons and plans to make and maintain behavioral changes.

Planning

When developing an educational strategy it is important to move from global, to general, to specific in the information hierarchy. The level of specificity must be carefully chosen based upon the content of the subject material, the amount of time, and the frequency of sessions available for covering it. While procedures usually must be taught with precision, cognitive and attitudinal education about a lengthy disease process, in which there will be ongoing contact with the patient, can be started in a very general way. With diabetes for example, cognitive material can be divided into survival skills, things the patient needs to know in order to live with the disease, and then the "nice-to-knows," which may improve outcomes but are less vital to survival. Home blood glucose monitoring and insulin administration (for those who require it) would be taught as survival skills.

It is important that your entire office have an educational focus, that there be plenty of educational materials and stimuli everywhere, and that all personnel from the receptionist through the most senior physician view themselves as educators (see chapter 7).

When talking with patients and their families it is important to look for openers that will facilitate where to start teaching. It also is helpful to prepare behavioral objectives which start where the learner is, focus on both the teacher and the learner, and are measurable so that outcomes can be evaluated. One of the most important planning tasks is to carefully prioritize short-term vs. long-term goals and to differentiate between the "need-to-knows" and "the nice-to-knows." The types of tools that will be used for teaching should be carefully chosen to meet the demands of the task at hand and the person who will be learning it.

Implementation

The many methods available to attain educational goals can be used individually or in combination, depending on the time line for the intervention, the setting where it occurs, learning styles, personnel needs, and costs. In general, the questions that should be asked are:

1) What method will be most acceptable to the patient and family?

2) What is the cost:benefit ratio in terms of time, personnel, start-up and continuing expense, and materials maintenance; and

3) How can you best get the attention of the learner and communicate the message most effectively?

The educational content should be tailored to the sociodemographic characteristics of the individual patient or target population. Criteria which must be considered include age, ethnicity/race, gender, educational level, and culture. Many people believe that learning is facilitated when information is transmitted by persons of similar sociodemographic or cultural background to the patient. Often, this is impossible. However attention can be paid to the style and language of the provider-patient interaction. Foreign-born patients, and those whose ethnic identity is with their country of origin, may be more comfortable talking about their health problems with a person who can communicate in their primary language. When patient and provider cannot be matched for language, it is helpful to have a trained interpreter or translation service, such as the AT&T language line, to assist with communications (Riddick, 1999). In the absence of a native speaking provider, teaching for chronic diseases and issues that will involve the family should include a family member or friend who speaks English and has an ongoing relationship with the patient whenever possible.

It is important to select the right strategy. Manner of presentation can have an important effect on how much the learner absorbs, and it is a good idea to avoid using inappropriate jargon. The amount of information and length of the teaching session must be consistent with the attention span of the patient at the time teaching occurs. Written materials should be at the correct reading level for the patient.

Teachable moments should be seized when they arise, even if they are out of priority order. Reinforcement of education by the various professionals involved in care is an important adjunct. A clinical pathway or teaching plan is important to facilitate all teachers conveying the same information.

Family members or friends become important adjuncts for people with special educational needs, such as individuals with developmental disabilities, especially those who cannot read or easily understand what is being said. If the individual lives in an institution or group home, staff members assume these functions. If possible, the same staff person should accompany the patient to all medical visits, and he or she should be made responsible for seeing that other staff members know what has to be done, why it is needed, and how to do it.

Evaluation

Evaluation of the educational intervention provides feedback to the patient, family, and professional on the success of teaching. It need not be formal; assessment of mastery is the important thing. Methods which can be used for evaluation include:

1) questioning the patient to assess verbal understanding of what has been taught;

2) having the patient or family demonstrate that he or she has learned the proper procedure or technique;

3) brief problem-solving cases or scenarios;

4) follow-up telephone calls from the provider or a staff member to determine whether further educational intervention is needed;

5) review of self-monitoring logs or diaries to determine adherence;

6) objective assessments, such as measurement of cholesterol or HbA1c; and

7) assessment of patient and family satisfaction with both the educational content and the teacher.

Instructional Modalities

Modalities That Usually Are Provider-Initiated

One-to-One Counseling

One-to-one counseling is the most frequently employed educational method in patient care settings and home environments. It may not be the most efficient or cost-effective method for the health care practitioner, but it is most effective for the individual learner. In this modality, a professional who is comfortable communicating without prejudice can develop a trusting relationship and teach about highly sensitive matters such as HIV or fertility control. The practitioner needs to be able to share information in an environment that is private and with limited interruption. Empathy and the ability to elicit questions are essential for useful counseling. Possible solutions to health problems can be offered and referral to specific focus organizations or programs such as Alcoholics Anonymous, bereavement support groups, or worksite health promotion programs can be facilitated. Major resources that are available in most communities are found in Chapter 3.

Group Teaching Support Groups

Group teaching support groups are very effective ways to meet the needs of congruent groups of patients because they teach and provide peer support simultaneously. Information can be imparted to a number of patients and their families at one time, and learning is increased in an informal environment. Patients can identify with one another and, as the cohesiveness of the group develops, its participants support and encourage one another. Learning is enhanced through group participation. Since individuals tend to conform to group norms and expectations concerning medical regimens, this process can powerfully facilitate attitude and behavior change (Lewis, 1984). Further, when group members interact with and support each other, stress can be reduced, and the incentive to change is facilitated (Teplitz, Egenes, & Brask, 1990). Group teaching is an excellent medium for diabetes education.

The major disadvantage of groups is that they sometimes mix people without adequate consideration of each individual's readiness or willingness to participate. Group teaching should be an adjunct to individualized instruction, and never should be substituted for the one-on-one component (Finkelmeier, 1995).

If patients can be appropriately grouped providers might consider having their own groups on topics for which there is sufficient demand. Even if reimbursement cannot be obtained, groups will be more cost-effective than continuous one-on-one teaching, particularly in the case of core content material for disease management.

Peer Education

Peer education can take two forms which may overlap. In the most frequent application, patients and their families who have faced specific problems are used to share their experience and expertise with others in similar situations. For example, individuals with HIV or AIDS frequently become the mentors of newly diagnosed patients and sometimes even teach primary prevention to at-risk patients; women who have undergone mastectomies for breast cancer visit new patients in a program called "Reach to Recovery," sponsored by the American Cancer Society. Many colleges use specially trained peer educators to teach human sexuality and sex education.

Peer educators also can be members of the same culture as the patients they are teaching. Often, they are individuals who are recruited from a specific community and trained to do outreach and teaching with members of their communities who have similar problems. We believe that peer educators could be very useful in the management of cardiovascular risk factors, smoking cessation, and prevention of substance abuse among other problems.

Other Media for Conveying the Message

Printed Materials

Brochures, information sheets, or flyers can be used alone or to reinforce information or skills attainment following an interaction with an individual health practitioner or a group session. Materials that combine text with visual cues, such as simple illustrations and photographs are more effective than detailed text.

In selecting appropriate printed materials, attention should be paid to the needs of the individual learner or target group with respect to language, literacy level, racial and ethnic sensitivity, gender identification, and those who are disempowered due to economic or educational disadvantage (Doak, Doak, & Root, 1996; Root, 1990). It is a good idea to pretest brochures and pamphlets prior to incorporating them into practice. This can be accomplished by having small groups of patients participate in focus groups, or by asking individual patients to compare and contrast the information in a variety of pamphlets and provide honest feedback.

Audiovisual Methods

Audiovisuals include audiotapes, films, passive or interactive videos, slide-tape shows, photographs, and illustrations. These educational tools generally are developed by independent film-makers, departments of health, national health organizations, universities, pharmaceutical companies, or community-based health consortia. Catalogs and listings of these resources are available in public and professional libraries and directly from the producers (See Chapter 3). While these instruments can peak interest in a subject, for the most part they are not interactive, and should be augmented by a discussion with a health care provider or educator or members of a peer network. Unless accompanied by coordinated printed material, audiotapes depend upon individual retention of information for later reflection. However, with the widespread use of home VCRs, this effect can be mitigated by giving patients copies of the tapes to take home and re-review at their convenience as needed. This approach also will allow families to be involved in the instructional process.

Videotapes can be used in clinic waiting rooms, examining rooms, conference/consultation rooms, or at home. They are especially useful for teaching procedure-oriented material, such as blood glucose monitoring technique, insulin administration, or breast self-examination. Adolescent medicine clinics and family planning clinics have made good use of this medium to explain reproductive physiology and the use of various contraceptive methods.

Audiotapes are a good medium for visually challenged and low literacy patients, and they provide an inexpensive way to reach individuals when printed information is not available in their primary language. They can be listened to via telephone, sent home with patients, and, with headsets, they can be used in private offices and clinic waiting areas (Root, 1990). Their low cost and convenience allow topics to be updated quickly. Benchmarks of good audiotapes are that they contain accurate information, are of high technical quality, brief, easily understood, use simple language, and are presented with well differentiated voices. Native speakers can present the material in their own dialects, including those for which there is no written language. Tapes can be used in conjunction with pamphlets, or the contents of a pamphlet can be read onto a tape. They can be made interactive by asking questions and instructing the listener to turn off the tape and then play the recorded answer after the question has been answered.

Interactive Methods

Audiotapes, videotapes, film strips, and computers can all be used as interactive media. Recently, technology-driven methods have been advanced, but limited economic status and fear of this new technology can present daunting barriers or obstruct participation. For those with sufficient skills, computer games and CD-ROM formats are a creative approach to patient education which younger people find particularly inviting. This format allows patients to learn at their own pace and to focus on topics which are of special interest to them.

For example, The New York State Department of Health created an interactive computer CD-ROM program targeted to sexually active young adults and adolescents. "Condomsense" addressed HIV/AIDS topics such as routes of transmission, risk-reduction strategies, and behaviors.

Many voluntary health organizations, coalitions of community-based organizations and departments of health, often in co-sponsorship, have created educational packages which combine techniques. The National Cancer Institute's Cancer and Diet Intervention project, "WIN At Home," combines risk-reduction materials that build upon one another and reinforce health behaviors.

Multimedia Methods

One example of a program targeted to native Americans was developed by the Native American AIDS Prevention Center and Human Health Organization, with consultation from the Centers for Disease Control and Prevention. The "We Owe It to Ourselves and to Our Children" multimedia approach incorporates three components: an illustrated book of poems and stories which reflects the groups' values, customs, and language presented in native storytelling format; an 8-minute videotape of the same name, narrated by native American health professionals, which uses native American characters and images from their lore; and two packets, *Understanding STDs and Understanding HIV and AIDS*, with pages of visuals from the video. These visuals with brief health messages at the bottom can be used to reinforce the video or individual educational messages (Rush & Capello, 1990). This example also highlights the importance of looking for resources, because materials you would not expect often exist.

Shared Decision-Making Programs

Shared decision-making provides patients and their families with general information about their conditions along with unbiased descriptions of the potential benefits and risks of the various surgical and nonsurgical treatments available to them (Kasper, Mulley, & Wennberg, 1992). A patient is referred to one of the programs using prespecified eligibility criteria for each program. Then, using information entered into the computer by the patient, such as age, symptom status, and medical history, patient-specific probabilities of the outcomes of each treatment alternative are presented. Video interviews with patients who have experienced the benefits and/or risks provide patients facing specific treatment decisions with a clear understanding of the possible outcomes in candid, human terms. Patients can control how much and what kind of information they receive. The developers are aware that some patients may find some information, such as cancer survival rates, disturbing, particularly if they have just learned of a diagnosis. To respect these situations, patients can first view information regarding their condition, and then proceed to other menu choices to select topics by either clicking a mouse or touching the screen.

The design and content of each program is based on extensive review and analysis of the published literature as well as on interviews with clinical investigators who care for patients. Great care is taken to assure that the programs will provide accurate and balanced presentations in a manner that is sensitive to the needs of patients.

The Internet—A Growing Resource Used by Both Parties

The Internet can be a valuable medium by which information can be exchanged with colleagues and patients. For those who have computers, the Internet is a readily available and constantly expanding source of information. It allows professionals to exchange information among themselves and with patients, and it provides access to information and support groups for patients and their families. While a recent survey reported that only 2% of consumers use the Internet as a primary source of medical information (Johnson, 1998), this figure is bound to grow over both the short and long run.

This medium is attractive to both patients and providers for a number of reasons. In addition to being a high-speed and often entertaining vehicle, which offers the user a great deal of variety and diversity, the Internet allows the user to search at his or her convenience 24 hours a day.

Communication is totally anonymous, and it costs nothing except the monthly Internet service provider charge.

Individuals can obtain information from four sources over the Internet: Websites, newsgroups, listservs, and electronic house calls/bulletin boards. Newsgroups are Internet-based forums for exchange of information on specific topics. They differ from online chat rooms in that they consist of a series of messages posted for other group members to see and comment upon if they want. Listservs are mailing lists that are designed to serve the needs of groups of people who want to exchange information on a common topic of interest. The same information is sent to everyone on the list via email, and comments can be returned to all members on the list.

Computer or voice bulletin boards offer a variety of services for patient education and counseling that patients can use from home. Electronic bulletin boards allow people to communicate by posting messages that can be read and responded to by others who have access to the board. Computer bulletin boards have made it possible to provide information and interpersonal support to a variety of populations in a cost effective manner. This is asynchronous communication in which participants do not talk directly to each other. Electronic bulletin boards are a popular feature of the Internet. In addition to education, they are a useful means of support for patients and their families, especially those with chronic diseases such as cancer and AIDS. Their advantages include the ability to allow participants to share information and solve problems of common interest without having to arrange time to attend face-to-face support groups; they allow participants to ask questions and receive answers from health professionals; and they let other users read or listen to these questions and answers. Thus participants benefit from hearing others' stories and concerns and how health professionals respond to them. Finally, electronic bulletin boards provide access to a library of expert information, such as books or pamphlets, on topics related to health care problems. Such easy accessibility reduces the frustration of searching for health information or waiting for agencies to forward material.

One example of a computer bulletin board is the Comprehensive Health Enhancement Support System (CHESS). Originally developed for breast cancer patients by Gustafson and colleagues (1993) at the University of Wisconsin, the CHESS program offers users 10 services relating to breast cancer:

1) "Question and answer," which answers the 250 questions most commonly asked by women with breast cancer;

2) "Instant library" with 150 articles on breast cancer-related issues;

3) "Getting help, with guidance on how to be an informed consumer;

4) "Referral directory," which lists organizations that will help to find services;

5) "Personal stories" of women sharing breast cancer experiences;

6) "Ask an expert," where users can leave confidential messages and receive confidential answers from medical experts;

7) "Discussion group" where users can leave messages on a bulletin board for other users to read and respond;

8) "Decision aid," which helps women decide among treatment options;

9) "Action plan," which helps women develop plans to implement their decisions; and

10) "Dictionary" which contains definitions of health-related terms.

Research on the use of CHESS shows that even older users quickly master the program, that it is used most frequently just after diagnosis and during treatments, and that the "discussion group" service is the most frequently used part of the program. Quality of life has been shown to improve as a result of the program (Gustafson et al., 1993). However, CHESS, in common with most electronic bulletin board programs, requires that both managers and users have computers. Consequently its applicability is limited to households with personal computers and to institutions or organizations with ongoing financial commitment to fund and maintain computer access.

Both the telephone- and computer-based bulletin boards have the potential to reinforce problem-solving learning and its use among family caregivers. Bulletin boards can provide expert information that caregivers need, and they can include programs that guide the user in developing plans. The question and answer group and discussion group formats enable professionals to encourage and guide the use of an orderly problem-solving approach. However, the impact of this technology on problem-solving behavior will depend on how it is used and guided by health care professionals.

Telephone and computer-based bulletin boards are efficient ways of helping family caregivers solve problems because professionals can listen and respond to questions or discussions at their convenience, and communication is managed automatically by computer programs. The fact that people can communicate anonymously at times of their choosing makes these programs attractive for many users.

Finally, entire manuals written for patients and families are available on the Internet. One example is the *Home Care Guide for Advanced Cancer* (Houts et al., 1997) which can be downloaded without charge. The authors of that particular work are available via e-mail to answer questions and refer readers to additional resources.

Who Posts the Information?

Information is put up on the Internet by a number of sources, among them government, voluntary health agencies, medical societies, universities, and individuals. Healthfinder (www.healthfinder.gov) is a filter for online health information created by the Federal Department of Health and Human Services. It provides links to health information from government health agencies, public health and professional groups, universities, support groups, medical journals and some news sites. Healthfinder also provides information about ongoing clinical trials for cancer and AIDS. The site can be searched by subject.

Quality of the Information

For all practical purposes, the Internet is an unregulated industry, in which anyone can put up anything they want. However, some voluntary efforts are being made to assure the quality of the information and establish criteria. Healthfinder, for example, evaluates health Web pages by looking at the credibility of the host institution, the individuals behind the site, the sponsors, and the originality and currency of the information.

Quackwatch (www.quackwatch.com) tries to ferret out and expose charlatan sites and point out errors in good sites, including the pages to which they link. Finally, the Health on the Net Foundation, which is based in Geneva, provides guidelines to differentiate credible sites from dubious ones and offers voluntary accreditation to those who are willing to abide by strict standards and a strong code of ethics. Awards are given to especially high-quality sites by credible medical organizations such as the AMA. Viewers can look for the HON logo.

Patient-Initiated Sources

Mass Media

For many individuals the news media are the major avenues to the health information which affects their health beliefs and behaviors. In a survey conducted by the National Health Council in the fall of 1997, 50% of respondents said they pay "a moderate amount" and 25% said they pay a "great deal" of attention to medical and health news reported by the media. That same survey found that more individuals rely on television (40%) than on their physicians (36%) as their primary source of health news, while 35% rely on magazines and journals and 16% on newspapers (Johnson, 1998). Fifty-eight percent of the survey respondents reported they had taken some action or changed their behavior as a result of having seen, heard, or read something in the media, and 42% said they sought further information as a result of media reports. Forty-five percent of those surveyed reported that discussing media reports with their physicians improved their relationships with their physicians (Johnson, 1998).

The media can provide immediate access to medical research findings by simplifying studies simultaneously reported in professional journals, albeit sometimes at the cost of sensationalism. Television has the potential to reach more people than any other medium. Messages are targeted by demographics, including spoken language, age and sex, even reaching illiterate or low-literacy groups (Lichter & Lichter, 1988; Nielsen Company, 1991).

Radio is even more accessible than television, and can be used in more venues, among them the car, on the beach and, more frequently, at work. Stations and broadcasts are targeted to specific audiences; teen pregnancy messages can accompany rock music, or osteoporosis can be discussed in a women's news-magazine format. Endorsement of the message comes from the use of respected disc jockeys or talk show hosts. Radio has been especially successful in engaging adolescents by call-in shows, such as San Francisco's "Street Soldiers," which is geared to discussion of adolescent problems in urban environments with special attention to drug use, health problems, and violence (Givahn, 1992).

Hardly a day goes by without some controversial and often contradictory news about some disease appearing in the newspaper, on television, radio, or in a magazine. While we strive to have patients and their families well-educated, it is important for both patients and providers to be somewhat critical of "new" studies and findings. Often, the data reported are very preliminary, and the statistical methods employed may be subject to question. Physicians frequently are flooded by telephone calls the day a news story appears, often before they are able to read the article in the news, let alone in the scientific journals. An important facet of educating patients is to have them carefully note new developments, and then discuss them with the physician, if appropriate, after the findings can be brought into perspective. Patients need to be instructed not to discontinue an otherwise important medication or therapy without such discussion.

Conclusion

The strategies of patient education discussed in this chapter are in keeping with the paradigm shift from total professional control of health care to shared responsibility with the patient and family. As individuals and families become more responsible for their own health maintenance, they reach out for knowledge about the details of managing chronic illness and seek ways to modify their risk factors. Every health care professional has a role to play in meeting this need for effective health education, and there is a place for every known educational medium. When selecting a teaching modality it is helpful to remember the following caveat:

"People remember . . . 10% of what they read; 25% of what they hear; 45% of what they see; 65% of what they hear and see; 70% of what they say and write, and 90% of what they say as they perform a task."

Chapter 3

Information Resources for Patient Education

Julia A. Bucher

Many providers, patients, and their families are unaware of or do not fully understand the community-based services that are available to help them learn more about illnesses, how to manage them, and how to cope. To aid in this task, we have compiled a list of resources that are available in most communities. The list is far from exhaustive, and readers are advised to consult other resources, including their local Yellow Pages. The directory is subdivided into two categories: voluntary national health organizations, and local community health agencies.

Medical staff can recommend that families learn about available educational services and resources before problems arise. They can stock helpful brochures and booklets in their offices, hand them out, run videos in the waiting room, loan out videos and books, give families phone numbers to call community resources for more information, and advertise local educational seminars and support/information groups. With this type of specific guidance, patients and families are more likely to do a more comprehensive job of learning about the disease and its management, especially when they are not under pressure to deal with a serious problem or crisis. If they need these educational resources later, they will know what to do and where to go immediately for more information.

---

*Note: The section on the National Hemophilia Association was written by Susan Resnik. The section on Internet Resources was compiled by William B. Bateman and Kimberly S. Glassman.

These community resources can supply health care practitioners with excellent written material for patient distribution. They also can assist the entire family in locating additional information, borrowing educational videos, and finding local educational seminars and support groups.

It would be imprudent to assume that physicians, nurses, and social workers are able to take care of all of a family's educational needs related to disease management and healthy coping. Educational resources from major organizations are constantly being updated and improved. In addition, local libraries provide links to written literature and audiovisual material from other organizations and publishers, and information clearinghouses can help patients and families find difficult-to-locate educational resources. Physicians and staff in managed care can inventory the educational material they are offering patients and families, update their stock, and refer families to these community resources.

This chapter discusses health education resources that are available in most communities and those services that link families to information about important community services, such as respite care, transportation, meals, visiting nurses, home hospice care, and paying medical or hospital expenses.

National Voluntary Organizations

American Heart Association

The American Heart Association (AHA) has a broad array of print and video educational materials for patient distribution. Their latest set of material for patients and families, "Answers By Heart," includes two-sided information sheets written in easy-to-read language. This material covers topics and conditions such as: angina, aphasia, arrhythmia, atrial fibrillation, high blood cholesterol and triglycerides, heart attack, heart disease, heart failure, high blood pressure, stroke, and transient ischemic attacks. The sheets include information on warning signs of these conditions as well as tips for recovery. "Answers By Heart" also teaches patients about diagnostic procedures such as echocardiography, electrophysiologic tests, and stress tests, and includes information on standard medical treatments such as coronary angiography, coronary angioplasty, anticoagulant and antiplatelet agents, coronary bypass surgery, heart valve surgery, carotid endarterectomy, cholesterol-lowering medicine, defibrillators, post heart surgery, high blood pressure medicine, pacemakers, and cardiac rehabilitation. "Answers By Heart" also summarizes important information on lifestyle and risk-reduction behaviors, which can be used by all types of patients. This subset of information instructs families on how to lower high cholesterol, cook healthy, eat a low-fat diet, eat out healthy, limit sodium, exercise, read food labels, reduce high blood pressure, quit smoking, manage stress, monitor weight and blood pressure, and lose weight. "Answers By Heart" can be ordered by calling 1-800-AHA-USA1 (1-800-242-8721). Selected topics also are available in Spanish, as are AHA's other patient education booklets and books, such as *The Healthy Walking Book.*

Cardiac education for patients also is available in a video series of 18 programs on topics about cardiology procedures, cardiovascular fitness, and cardiovascular wellness. These videos average 10 to 12 minutes in length and are available in English and Spanish. Other films and videos also are available for patient education.

The AHA is also the major provider of information about stroke. The AHA Stroke Connection at 1-800-553-6321 offers national newsletters, stroke education materials, and other resources, such as information on how to organize stroke clubs. They also sponsor Mended Hearts, groups for heart surgery patients, and provide guidelines on how to organize these groups.

All materials described above can be ordered by health professionals or directly by patients and their families by contacting the AHA. Check the local telephone book and request a list of resources and order form.

American Cancer Society, National Cancer Institute, and Cancer Care, Inc.

The American Cancer Society (ACS) distributes patient and family education material on cancer prevention, treatment, and coping. Booklets and videos are available in English and Spanish for different age groups. Prevention topics include information on how to perform breast and testicular self-exams; when to get specific cancer checkups; why to avoid tanning and sun exposure; how to quit smoking; what to eat; and what to know in general about many types of cancer in men, women, and children. A wide variety of literature and material is available on the effects of smoking cigarettes, chewing tobacco, and passive smoke. In addition, medical treatment is explained for many types of cancer such as malignant melanoma, bladder, brain, breast, colorectal, esophagus, larynx, lung, ovarian, and prostate cancer. Questionable methods of treatment are listed. Finally, information on coping, such as managing ostomies, dealing with depression, understanding issues of sexuality, and coping with survivors' issues, is available, and the ACS sponsors groups that provide education, such as "I Can Cope" for all types of cancers; "Man to Man" for prostate cancer; or "Reach to Recovery" for women who undergo surgery for breast cancer.

Similar to the AHA, the ACS also has literature for professionals and community leaders on running self-help groups and conducting community screenings and cancer risk assessments.

Material can be ordered by calling 1-800-ACS-2345 and requesting an order form list. Information specialists who answer these calls also will send out material specific to patient and family requests and needs, such as general information on the right to cancer pain relief and local information on financial assistance options for diagnostic tests.

The American Cancer Society works closely with another important cancer education resource, the Cancer Information Service (CIS), a national information and education network of the National Cancer Institute, which is the nation's primary agency for cancer research. The CIS publishes educational material, some of which is written for audiences with as low as a 5th-grade reading level. In addition, the CIS 800 number puts patients and families in touch with databases and technical journal articles that report the latest information on treatment options. The Cancer Information Service (reached at 1-800-4-CANCER) answers questions about cancer in English or Spanish, informs patients about community resources, and mails publications and brochures to patients' homes.

Cancer Care, Inc., a social service agency with offices in a number of states, also provides patient education materials. Social workers take the calls, mail information to callers, and publicize teleconferences in which patients and families can listen to physicians and health care staff talk about specific cancers and coping strategies. During these educational teleconferences, callers have the opportunity to ask questions and discuss issues with a large listening audience. Cancer Care, Inc. can be reached by dialing 1-800-813-HOPE (4673).

American Diabetes Association

Information on diabetes can be ordered by calling 1-800-DIABETES. Many new booklets have been printed to assist diabetics and their families to manage type 1 and type 2 diabetes and improve the quality of their lives. For example, the booklet "Carbohydrate Counting" is available at three levels of complexity to help meet the needs of different patients, and one of the new books, titled *Managing Diabetes On A Budget*, teaches families how to comparison-shop for supplies and medications and get the most benefit from their insurance coverage. Material from the ADA covers needs of mature as well as new diabetics, helping them identify and interpret patterns in blood glucose levels.

The latest teaching series, "Life With Diabetes," was developed by the Michigan Diabetes Research and Training Center for use by health professionals. It presents a comprehensive curriculum for diabetic education, instructor notes, and an evaluation and documentation plan. Contact the ADA for order forms for publications, teaching series, and a long list of audiovisual rentals and purchases.

American Lung Association

The American Lung Association has a wide range of educational materials in English and Spanish on asthma, chronic obstructive pulmonary disease, tuberculosis, occupational lung disease, other adult and pediatric lung disease, environmental health, and smoking and health. Materials in print, film and video, are available for public, patient, and school health education and can be obtained by calling 1-800-LUNG-USA (1-800-586-4872).

Arthritis Foundation

The catalog of educational materials for patients from the Arthritis Foundation divides topics into two categories. Disease-specific topics include information about causes, symptoms, diagnosis, and treatments for: ankylosing spondylitis; arthritis and inflammatory bowel disease; back pain; Behcet disease, bursitis, tendinitis, and other soft-tissue rheumatic syndromes; carpal tunnel syndrome; CPPD (crystal deposition disease); Ehlers-Danlos syndrome; fibromyalgia; gout; infectious arthritis; lupus; Lyme disease; Marfan syndrome; myositis; osteoarthritis; osteogenesis imperfecta; osteonecrosis; osteoporosis; Paget disease; polyarteritis nodosa and Wegner granulomatosis; polyalgia rheumatica and giant cell arteritis; pseudoxanthoma elasticum; psoriatic arthritis; Raynaud phenomenon; reflex sympathetic dystrophy syndrome; Reiter syndrome; rheumatoid arthritis; sarcoidosis; scleroderma; and Sjogren syndrome.

Medication topics include information on aspirin and other nonsteroidal anti-inflammatory drugs, corticosteroids, gold treatment, hydroxychloroquine (Plaquenil), methotrexate, penicillamine (Cuprimine, Depen), a drug guide from *Arthritis Today*, and information on using new medicines wisely. Several of these booklets are printed in Spanish.

In addition, booklets are available on other arthritis-related topics, such as arthritis and employment; pregnancy; children; diet; activities; exercise; fatigue; pain; stress; surgery; lab tests; and health plans. A number of videos are included in the list.

The National Hemophilia Foundation (NHF)

The NHF, located at 116 West 32nd Street New York, NY (phone 212-328-3700), serves as a pivot for communication, providing advocacy and support for persons with hemophilia and their families throughout the United States. Founded in 1948, this national organization continues to be dedicated to finding the cure for inherited bleeding disorders and to preventing and treating the complications of these disorders.

Publications include a wealth of educational pamphlets and videotapes on various aspects of the illness, a model educational tool, "The Patient/Family Model," and printed newsletters. Discussion of research and practice issues for physicians, nurses, social workers and physical therapists are also addressed in specific publications. The NHF's Medical and Scientific Advisory Council (MASAC), a multidisciplinary committee consisting of hemophilia treatment experts, disseminates information and shares research through these channels.

NHF has also established a clearinghouse providing information about the multiplicity of concerns involved in hemophilia and its complications, including HIV and hepatitis. It is called Hemophilia and AIDS/HIV Network for the Dissemination of Information (HANDI) 1-800-41-HANDI.

The Women's Outreach Network (WONN), The Men's Advocacy Network (MANN) and The Chapter Outreach Demonstration Project (CODP) provided the groundwork for PEER, a composite of WONN and MANN. Today these networks, already in place throughout the United States, can serve as extenders of peer education and outreach, collaborating with chapters, treatment centers and agencies.

The National Asthma Education and Prevention Program

The National Asthma Education and Prevention Program (NAEPP) is located at the National Institutes of Health (NIH), National Heart, Lung and Blood Institute. *Guidelines for the Diagnosis and Management of Asthma* is available through the NIH (publication No. 97-4053). A shortened version entitled *Practical Guide for the Diagnosis and Management of Asthma* (publication No. 97-4053) is also available.

Local Agencies

Area Agency on Aging

Nurses, social workers, and caseworkers at the local Area Agency on Aging provide patients and families with a wide range of educational materials. They can meet families in the home or office and give them detailed written information about health and social service entitlements and options for getting additional help at home. They also help families find the information they need on illnesses, and refer them to other important educational services in the local community.

Telephone numbers for staff at the local Area Agency on Aging, sometimes referred to as the Senior Center or Senior Services, can be located in the White Pages of the telephone book under "Area Agency on Aging." They also are listed in the Blue Pages under the same name in the County Services section. If these numbers are not listed, each state has a state Office of Aging listed in the blue pages under the State Services section. The Office of Aging will refer the caller to their local Area Agency on Aging office. Most counties have their own offices. Smaller or rural counties sometimes share an office among two or three counties.

Cooperative Extension Services

Another educational service that stocks excellent written material, but perhaps does not publicize itself as widely among health care professionals, is Cooperative Extension Services, which is sponsored by the United States Department of Agriculture. Extension agents (sometimes referred to as county agents) offer community education on issues related to family, health, and aging. They have offices in all counties and serve both urban and rural communities. Their written materials are reader-friendly and can be obtained by calling the local agent's office.

Health topics published for consumer distribution include excellent tips on nutrition, shopping wisely for groceries, preparing food safely at home, losing weight, and feeding children nutritiously. Other written material focuses on key safety issues and includes discussions of home environmental risk assessment, preventing water contamination by managing hazardous products safely, disposing of other hazardous household waste, and pest removal. Psychosocial topics include coping with loss, managing a life-threatening illness, and helping others manage.

Local Libraries and Information Clearinghouses

Local libraries can order pamphlets on disease prevention and management and usually offer an array of books and videos on different diseases. Patients and families can ask the library to obtain information for them.

Information and referral clearinghouses are agencies that specialize in helping families find community services. They have different titles in different communities or parts of the country. Some examples are the Office of Human Resources, United Way, religious agencies (such as Catholic Charities or the local Councils of Churches), and Community Mental Health Centers.

Usually accessed by telephone, staff members are experienced in helping families find help from other community agencies and volunteer groups, as well as information from organizations such as those listed above. The telephone book is a starting place to locate this type of resource. Most local telephone books contain a special section, sometimes referred to as the "Guide to Human Services" section, that lists community agencies and the services they provide. Often, this section is printed on colored paper to set it off from the rest of the directory. Frequently, the pages are blue. Look at the table of contents in the beginning of the local telephone book for the Guide to Human Services—or a similar title.

Internet Resources

There are many sites on the World Wide Web where health professionals can obtain educational information for their patients. Hundreds, if not thousands of health information resources are available on the Internet, but without quality control. The October 21, 1998 theme issue of *JAMA* (the *Journal of the American Medical Association*) explores this topic. A brief annotated list of some sites that we find interesting follows.

Common professional sites such as Medscape (www.medscape.com) offer a "one-stop shop" for both professional and patient information. Medscape provides direct links to resource databases such as Medline, as well as weekly highlights of the latest scientific and medical information from medical journals. Medscape News provides a selection called "What your patients are reading." This site lists lead articles from the press that may have caught the interest of the public, and thus may be a source of interest or concern for patients. A section titled "Patient Resources" provides links to reputable publications from government agencies, such as the National Institute on Aging's publication *High Blood Pressure: A Common but Controllable Disorder*. These materials can be ordered from the agencies online, or alternatively, can be printed for patients' use. One drawback to printing for immediate use is the small font used in these materials. A better choice for practices with large elderly populations would be to download the materials for reformatting in a word processing program. This allows use of the material in a customized format for elders or patients with reduced vision.

"Patient Page" from the Journal of the American Medical Association (accessible at www.ama-assn.org) is available both at the website and in the weekly journal. Each issue features patient education materials for a common health problem. The website offers clinicians the advantage of reviewing the variety of topics that can be printed for patients. These Patient Pages are easy-to-read, one- or two-page documents. Some contain graphics to reinforce the printed information. They may be reproduced by clinicians for patient use at no cost.

Healthfinder (www.healthfinder.gov) offers materials from various federal agencies such as NIH and HRSA and website links to professional societies. Selecting a condition such as arthritis, provides a direct link to the "Arthritis Foundation" (www.arthritis.org) home page, where professionals or patients can then obtain specific information about self-management.

Covering common disease areas, the American Heart Association (www.americanheart.org), the American Cancer Society (www.cancer.org), the Arthritis Foundation (www.arthritis.org), the American Lung Association (www.lungusa.org), and the American Diabetes Association (www.diabetes.org) all provide comprehensive information for both professionals and patients. These websites contain documents that can be downloaded and printed, or addresses for ordering materials online or by mail.

The American Academy of Family Physicians (AAFP) homepage (www.aafp.org) offers a link to "Health Information for Patients" which provides a variety of useful patient education materials. These include patient information handouts and "The AAFP Family Health and Medical Guide," a series of self-care and self-diagnosis flow charts, 22 of which are available online. Patient education brochures that answer "the most frequently-asked questions for many common health problems" are also available.

The U.S. Centers for Disease Control and Prevention (www.cdc.gov) and the U.S. Food and Drug Administration (www.fda.gov) are among the government sites offering useful material for patients. The CDC site provides information about prevention guidelines, health risks, and diseases. The FDA provides the latest information on foods, human and animal drugs, and cosmetics.

Some very interesting and comprehensive sites include Dr. Koop's Community (http://drkoop.com) and the Virtual Hospital (www.vh.org). These are offered by the former Surgeon General and the University of Iowa, respectively. Both are fun to explore and provide a wealth of consumer information on health promotion, disease prevention, living with diseases, and the health care system.

Finally, for those seeking interactive patient education software, resources exist like the University of Iowa's "Patient Education Institute" (www.patient-education.com). This homepage offers online demonstrations and ordering. Among other services, they offer customized health information software and CD-ROMs aimed at "reaching the widest audience, including the functionally illiterate and 'computer-illiterate' populations."

Summary

The intent of this chapter is to show that there are substantial community resources for patient education and support. The time and cost efficiencies demanded in today's health care environment make their use essential for optimal care delivery.

Chapter 4

Interdisciplinary Care Management and Collaborative Care

Kimberly S. Glassman and Kim Neall

Today, more than ever before, the healthcare environment requires a team approach to the delivery of patient care. The shift from illness to wellness, and the need to reduce the cost of care while maintaining quality, has made collaborative care management an essential component of healthcare delivery systems in both acute and community-based settings.

What Is Collaborative Care?

Collaborative care is defined as "inclusionary care . . . a condition of an accountable practice in which desired patient/family outcomes are the unifying force" (Zander, 1995, p. 1). It defines a need for all providers to work together in supporting patients and their families through their acute hospitalization, or helping them to live with chronic conditions by maximizing their ability to care for themselves. While all disciplines recognize a need to work collaboratively, all work environments require systems to avoid conflict and support collaboration among these providers. Tools such as critical pathways help to identify more clearly the role that each provider plays in moving patients toward the desired outcomes. In this chapter, the concepts of care and case management, integrated care,

49

and disease management will be considered as examples of collaborative care.

Integration of care among all provider settings is necessary to establish a seamless continuum of care. Ideal integration involves a comprehensive array of providers who are linked together to provide appropriately accessed health care services. Bringewatt (1995) identifies a "trinocular" approach to integration of care for people with chronic diseases, who are so poorly served by today's "component" approach to care. The "trinocular" view describes the perspectives of the three professional groups that are likely to shape the delivery of chronic care: acute care, long-term care and managed care.

Acute care is organized around the notion of illness, and solutions are directed toward a cure. It is high-tech, short-term, and episodic, and uses highly trained professionals. Long-term care professionals view chronic care in terms of function, and solutions are focused on care options. It is ongoing, and uses paraprofessionals and families as key providers. Managed care professionals tend to view chronic care in terms of optimizing health through primary, secondary, and tertiary prevention. They are concerned with educating people about the impact of lifestyles on health and well being over the long term. All three perspectives must be integrated to achieve quality and control health care costs.

Collaborative care commonly is operationalized by two key methodologies: case management and critical pathways (Zander, 1995, p. 19). Case management can be described as a system that focuses the accountability of an individual or group for:

- Coordinating a patients' care across an episode (hospitalization) or continuum;
- Ensuring and facilitating the achievement of quality and clinical cost outcomes;
- Negotiating, procuring, and coordinating services and resources needed by the patient/family;
- Intervening at key points or variances for individual patients;
- With collaborative teams, addressing and resolving patterns in aggregate variances that have a negative impact on quality and cost;
- Creating opportunities to enhance outcomes (Zander, 1995)

Nurses have a long history of involvement in case management. The community health model used a case management model to care for patients and families over time. Insurance companies instituted case management as a way to control costs of catastrophic claims while ensuring quality (More & Mandell, 1997). In recent years, it has been used in hospital settings to decrease length of stay, thus decreasing the cost of the hospital episode.

There are many ways to structure accountability for case management. In the hospital setting, clinical nurses may serve as case managers. Primary nurses may serve as the care managers for their patients, but many hospitals employ advanced practice nurses to coordinate care to a population of patients during the entire hospital episode. These nurse case managers coordinate care for patients from admission through discharge; they may conduct preoperative classes to prepare patients for surgery, and teach post-hospital care. Utilization case management typically uses nurses trained in utilization review to audit care processes and patient placement. These nurses also may perform a discharge-planning function, but they may not be involved in the direct provision of care, such as patient and family education. Some hospitals are beginning to explore ways to combine these two different groups of nurses to perform a more comprehensive form of care management, which both manages the clinically complex patient and monitors resource consumption in less complicated patients through the use of tools such as pathways (Zander, 1995).

The importance of the interdisciplinary team is paramount in all collaborative care management systems. Hospital staff familiar with collaboration between nurses, doctors, social workers, and therapists are aware of the fragmentation that exists among providers, which often results from cumbersome communication systems. The hospital-based case manager facilitates timely communication among all members of the team, particularly with patient and family, to ensure that care occurs without delay, thus meeting the goal of decreased length of stay. The health plan case manager works with the provider to address nonmedical issues and coordinate care and patient satisfaction. Because HMOs link the financial and service delivery components so closely, health plan case management can be a more effective tool to control resource utilization than in most other case management settings (Hicks, 1993).

Collaborative Care Models in the Community

Outpatient collaborative care programs serve a variety of populations, and often are shaped by social problems, health concerns, and other factors (Moxley, 1994). Historically these programs have used innovative, integrated approaches to provide care for people whose social problems might cause them to access the health system in more costly ways. People with substance abuse or chronic conditions such as HIV can be managed in community-based case management programs, such as AID Atlanta, which coordinates a variety of disciplines including nursing, social work, therapists, and pastoral care to provide multidisciplinary expertise based on the need of the patient (Sowell & Meadows, 1994). A community-focused case management system at Carondelet St. Mary's Hospital and Health Center uses nurses as both coordinators and providers of care (Satinsky, 1995). These case managers work within an ambulatory network of several community health centers. Patients may be referred to the case management system from any provider in the health system. The most prevalent groups of patients are those with chronic illnesses, acute care patients whose conditions have been exacerbated by chronic illnesses and who will return to baseline functioning, and patients facing the end of life. Close collaboration with patients is the hallmark of this model, as care is negotiated between the case manager and the patient.

Payer-based case managers may coordinate patients' care across several settings, usually addressing the needs of those with chronic or catastrophic illness. These programs may tailor care to assisting patients to access the healthcare system at the most effective point, and emphasize wellness and preventive measures, rather than waiting for severe symptoms to occur. One example of such programs is life care planning which outlines comprehensive care for the life of a patient with catastrophic injury, including medical and health costs, living expenses, transportation, mental health services, and other types of long-term expenses (Deutsch & Sawyer, 1990; Weed & Riddick, 1992).

As care managers, nurses played a key role in the evolution of disease management. Utilization review was an early focus of managed care organizations. Efforts were directed toward more closely managing and supervising care to obtain cost-effective results. The antagonistic nature of this approach served to polarize providers and payers, and led to the development of utilization management. Utilization management emphasized the use of clinical guidelines, often derived from utilization review process data, rather than academic guidelines, and assessed patients' disease states against internally established criteria. This phase of care management emphasized conformity, rather than evidence-based science, to structure care, and provided little opportunity for collaboration among providers, payers, or patients (Ward & Rieve, 1997). Case management offered a more proactive approach to care management, with nurses working collaboratively with physicians and interdisciplinary teams to develop care guidelines emphasizing evidence-based and regional best-practices to achieve a higher level of patient-centered care. However, these case management programs often were facility-based, and thus episodic in their approach to care management.

Disease management offers a more seamless, integrated system of care for a population of patients across a continuum. Zalta (1994) defines disease management as proactive case management. At its best, it includes "information-intensive series of clinical processes and services across the continuum of health care that identifies the medically at-risk population and professionally manages patients in a manner that improves care, promotes wellness and manages/reduces cost" (Ward & Rieve, 1997, p. 235).

There are many sources of guidance for developing disease management programs, and all identify some basic elements (Cohen, 1997; Todd & Nash, 1997). The first step in establishing a disease management program is to determine the populations to manage. Identification of at-risk members through triggers and risk profiles for the targeted diseases is essential for initiating the process of disease management. Once the key triggers of a disease have been determined, and the process for risk patients identified, health assessment and evaluation of the identified population can begin.

Case managers are critical to coordinating or providing these assessments, particularly for patients with chronic illnesses. Some disease management programs sponsor home visits to evaluate clinical and environmental risk factors in the home for their clients with asthma (Case Management Advisor, 1995). Determination of benefits is an important function for case managers in disease management programs. Payer plans are structured to control costs, yet the case manager often must advocate for exceptions to the usual payment. By negotiating wellness care, such as smoking cessation, diet, and exercise programs, up front, costly illness care may be avoided in the long run. Case managers also may coordinate development of pathways and disease management guidelines, which should be evidence-based, and use all available science to underpin the recommended care.

Care plan implementation in disease management programs requires commitments from all participants. Patients, families, and all providers must participate in the process of health maintenance, and case managers often are key to obtaining necessary buy-in from all parties. Administration of the plan is the responsibility of case managers. Patient and family education about the program, and assisting patients in self-management require that case managers direct their efforts toward improving patient outcomes in these areas. Case managers must be knowledgeable about each patient's level of participation and compliance with treatments, and they must be prepared to provide individualized education and counseling for those patients who are unable to adhere to their recommended program. Identifying these patients requires that the case manager be informed of triggers such as emergency room visits, and unplanned hospitalizations. Health plan case managers routinely search for these events through usual claims review. These triggers provide ongoing information which is essential to maintaining quality and controlling costs in disease management programs.

Compliance monitoring in the form of follow-up reminder telephone calls to patients to be sure they are taking their medications, have adequate supplies of drugs, and keep their clinic appointments can help ensure that patients with chronic illnesses are properly maintained. Program evaluation is required to ensure that disease management programs are indeed meeting the clinical and financial outcomes. Outcome measurement of clinical, satisfaction, and cost indicators along the continuum of care provided the feedback that disease management is a useful method of providing care.

There are many disease management programs underway, with promising preliminary results. Hypertension, with its broad impact on quality and cost of care, is a common target for disease management. Some early programs have demonstrated a need for significant buy-in from all levels of an organization to be successful (Christianson, Pietz, Taylor, Woolley, & Knutson, 1997).

The hypertension disease management program at Cedars-Sinai Medical Center in Los Angeles focused on this condition as a way to improve the health of a large number of patients. They are conducting a three-way study in which they are comparing (1) a low intensity intervention consisting of a physician alert; (2) a high-intensity intervention using a disease management clinic; and (3) a control group of patients enrolled in fee-for-service or HMO care (Weingarten, 1997). Patients receive baseline, 6-month and 12-month follow-up with tracking of intermediate outcomes such as blood pressure control, visit costs, and laboratory and drug costs. Interim results appear promising, with the disease management patients showing significantly improved outcomes in lowering of systolic blood pressure.

The role of the nurse case manager in development and implementation of these programs is expanding. The nurse-managed Lipid Clinic at the University of North Carolina (UNC) is one such example (Thomas, 1997). As part of the UNC cardiovascular risk reduction program, patients are referred to the lipid clinic for ongoing management of hyperlipidemia. The nurse case manager is responsible for enrolling new patients, education and counseling about cardiovascular risk factors, assisting patients to better manage their pharmacologic therapies, coordination with other health professionals, triaging patients to other services, and development of policies. The initial visit focuses on the need for treatment, medical and diet history, assessment of the need for pharmacologic therapy, and discussion of need for behavior changes. Follow-up appointments continue the theme of negotiating behavior change, with modifications in the treatment regimen. Payment for these preventive services remains problematic, with many health centers absorbing the cost of this follow-up care as part of the overall business package. Partnering with payers remains an option to be explored, particularly when clinical programs can demonstrate success in managing patients through the use of less costly resources.

Some employers have instituted case management programs for their employees, such as workers' compensation programs that help employees get back to work in temporary jobs that do not interfere with their injuries. Again, the wellness philosophy that underpins these programs emphasizes the importance of keeping the worker productive and contributing to the workplace.

Collaborative Care Management Tools

All collaborative care management programs require tools to coordinate and communicate plans of care to all providers. One common care management tool is an interdisciplinary clinical pathway. Clinical pathways can be developed across the continuum. In acute care settings, they outline the anticipated course of hospitalization, or recovery from illness across a timeline, with the specific care details listed for each involved discipline. The most useful pathways in acute care settings are physician-driven, and thus incorporate appropriate evidence-based practice guidelines into the plan of care. Delays in education and discharge planning occur when staff are unable to predict when a patient will be discharged. Physicians are unable to plan for discharge when diagnostic tests are delayed or results are unavailable. Having the physician's medical plan listed for other providers ensures that important aspects of a hospitalization, such as patient/family education and discharge planning, occur on time.

In the community setting, pathways help focus providers on the sequencing of care for a variety of chronic conditions, or wellness programs. These pathways may outline recommended patient/family teaching protocols that build a patient's knowledge base over a series of visits. Office visits may be supplemented with home visits or phone calls to ensure that patients are adhering to their prescribed treatments through supportive interventions.

There are several resources which describe the development of clinical pathways (Cohen & Cesta, 1997; Crawford-Swent, 1996). The development and implementation process is generally the same, regardless of the setting of care. The process used at NYU Medical Center, an academic medical center in New York City, included the support of senior administrators, as well as identifying key experts to facilitate the process (see Figure 4.1). A physician leader and a nurse administrator were chosen to work with groups of practicing physicians and other clinicians, in forums which identified best practice. A senior research scientist brought the available research to the work groups to reinforce a pathway's use of evidence-based practice. Where evidence was not strong, consensus of expert opinion was used. While some pathways, such as those for postoperative care, had strong agreement among practitioners, others, such as those for heart failure and other chronic illnesses, required a different approach. Internal clinical evaluation studies of NYUMC's patient population were required to determine the characteristics of this medical center's patients, and identify the subgroups that could fit established practice guidelines. By referencing established practice guidelines, such as those developed by the Agency for Health Care Policy and Research, the providers' attention was directed to addressing and recommending pre- and post-hospital care, in addition to inpatient management.

Anticipating a patient's recovery and the resultant care needed is the major utility of a pathway in reducing hospital length of stay. Clinical pathways also can address a continuum and link the care provided in the hospital to that required in the home, or follow-up visits in a clinic or office. As hospital stays have become shorter, providers in home care or

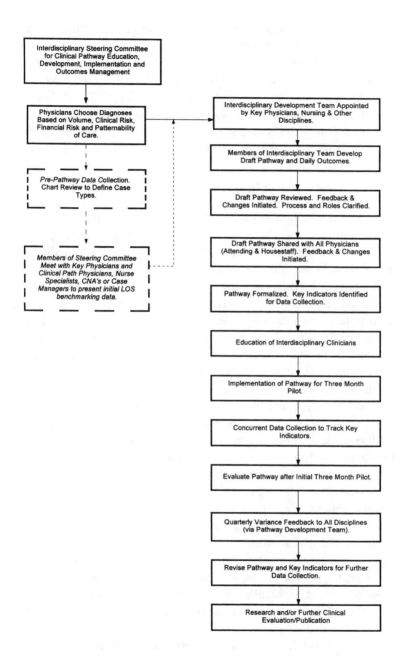

Figure 4.1 NYU Medical Center, Case Management and Clinical Pathways Program, Clinical Pathway Process.

community clinics need to be aware of the appropriate follow-up care, and the anticipated path for a patient's recovery after discharge. Pathways that include post-discharge care and outcomes are useful for focusing community nurses on the key complications, which may arise as more patients recuperate at home. These linkages between plans of care are important communication tools for hospital and community providers to remain informed about how individual patients are progressing toward recovery, and provide an opportunity to measure outcomes over time.

Evaluation of Care

Management of care requires evaluation of outcomes to determine success or areas for improvement. Clinical pathways that incorporate established, evidence-based practice guidelines provide the ability to track quality and outcomes of care. When this information can be used by the collaborative teams who created the pathway, practice changes and improved care can result. For example, a pathway or office-based guideline for heart failure would incorporate best-practice guidelines including the use of ACE inhibitors and the need to evaluate patients' ability to self-manage their condition, particularly the need to monitor weight. The number of patients meeting the guidelines can be tracked and, more importantly, those patients not meeting guidelines due to comorbidity or other clinical conditions can be studied for opportunities to improve care. Moreover, variance data from pathways can point to a need for systems improvements, such as delays in diagnostic tests or consistent recording of patient weights through home follow-up programs. The use of variance data to improve systems of care is one of the positive outcomes of care management. A negative outcome occurs when variance data are used to police care and stop or limit options without suggestions for improvement.

Evaluation of care is becoming a focus in all provider arenas. The Health Care Financing Administration, which administers the federal Medicare program, has supported home health agencies' use of an outcome measurement tool, OASIS, to measure their impact on patient outcomes over time (Shaughnessy, Crisler, Schlenker, & Arnold, 1997). These assessments, developed at the University of Colorado Center for Health Services Research, provide valuable information about patients' condition at entry into home care, at 60 days, and at discharge from home care services. Linking these outcome measures with those done on selected populations cared for in integrated health systems will provide comprehensive feedback about how we as providers are influencing patient outcomes over time and across settings.

Evaluation also can occur within integrated delivery systems. Nurses at Kaiser Permanente, Northern California Region, developed and implemented a patient outcomes measurement tool, the Health Status Outcomes Dimension (H-SOD), that is used to follow patients' health status in all settings—clinics, physicians' offices, acute and long-term care. Patient populations tracked include selected high-risk groups such as those with heart failure, joint replacements, and premature neonates (Lush, Henry, Foote, & Jones, 1997). The goal is to determine the predictive value of such a tool in identifying when patients' health status deteriorates and requires intervention.

Building Collaboration among Agencies

A unique example of ongoing collaborative care management is the Continuum of Care Program for heart failure (HF) patients at NYUMC. Responding to a need for hospital length-of-stay reduction, and an urgent need to provide better communication of patients needs across the continuum, NYUMC partnered with Visiting Nurse Service of New York (VNSNY) and the Division of Nursing at New York University (NYU) to expand a post-discharge follow-up program. NYUMC had developed an inpatient care management program, consisting of a pathway for patients with an uncomplicated exacerbation of their HF, a comorbidities pathway supplement for those patients whose HF was exacerbated by one of six major comorbidities, and a case management option for end-stage HF patients, those with multiple comorbidities, or new onset of failure with unknown etiology. The pathway task force, led by several cardiologists, was successful at reducing length of stay by identifying system improvements. A cardiology case manager provided post discharge follow-up through phone calls to those patients who were at risk for readmission.

Lacking in this earlier program, however, was a system to help prevent readmissions. The partnership between these agencies created the Continuum of Care Program which now provides a link between hospital and home by extending the case management into the community. Patients with HF are discharged with one of three options: phone calls from the cardiology case manager and adult nurse practitioner students from NYU; phone calls plus VNSNY, for those patients who require home care; and phone calls plus home care plus home visits from adult NP students, who provide individualized instruction in self-management of HF.

Through this program, funded by the United Hospital Fund in 1997, preliminary results have shown the heart failure readmission rate decreased by half, from 10.4 to 5.5 %, and the interval between readmissions increased from 8 weeks to 18 weeks (Glassman et al., 1998). Collaboration among providers and patients and their families has been a key factor in the early success of this program.

The future plans include the development of community supports through hospital-based outpatient programs, such as a heart failure center, providing clinical support to physicians' practices and wellness care for cardiac patients. Partnering with payers, particularly in a risk-sharing environment, will allow for some of these costs to be shared proportionately among all settings.

Collaboration with Patients and Families

Providing patients and families with the knowledge they need to carry out self-care is essential for acute care settings with shortened hospital stays, as well for community settings, where shortened clinic or decreased home care visits have become the norm. Acute care clinical pathways should identify the sequencing of the teaching, with an emphasis on what patients need to know to care for themselves during the recuperative phase. More detailed information on maintaining wellness could be discussed at a follow-up appointment with their provider. Since patients' learning in the hospital may be hampered by pain, etc., follow-up phone calls provide an opportunity for staff to answer their questions, or assess the need for additional learning once patients are in their home environments. Moreover, patients and their families can be reassured that despite a short hospital stay, assistance is available.

A patient version of the clinical pathway provides patients and families with an abbreviated plan of care. The patient pathways for hospitalized patients at NYUMC describe the key activities patients must do each day, such as the number of times/levels of respiratory exercises or distance to ambulate after surgery. This approach reinforces the need for patients to actively participate in their recovery and the activities which will facilitate such recovery. The patient pathways discuss the members of the interdisciplinary team, and the timing of their visits, such as social work or nutrition consultations, and also give the suggested date of discharge. This information is essential for patients and families to use when planning to return home. Family members may need to arrange for time off from work to help the patient return home. When the patient pathway is distributed in the surgeon's office as part of a preadmission packet, patients and families can be well prepared for their anticipated hospital course. Patient pathways for those with chronic illnesses can be designed for ambulatory or home care settings. These tools identify the learning sequence of self-care activities for patients in the hospital, and when they return home.

An interesting development in patient pathways is those that use symbols, rather than text. Designed for a multicultural population in Seattle, the patient pathways at the University of Washington Academic Medical Center use graphic elements and icons to communicate care to this culturally diverse population (Nemeth et al., 1998). Patients and staff developed the pathway content, and the icons were validated by cross-cultural populations (Figure 4.2). In health care settings where patient's literacy level or language may be barriers to learning, "picture pathways" can be useful tools to impart information.

Partnerships to Promote Collaborative Care

Collaborative care management can benefit patients and providers by communicating the plan of care to all involved patients, families, payers, and providers. Such clarity of communication allows all providers to be accountable for the care they are most qualified to give, and avoids duplication or gaps in service. Building relationships among these parties is necessary to achieve integrated care management. Consumers, providers, and payers need to participate in collaborative arrangements for quality outcomes and cost efficiencies to be achieved. An overarching concern remains about payment for health care services, as much of our reimbursement system is still based on an illness model of care, where preventive services are not reimbursed. Collaboration among providers and payers can greatly benefit the recipients of care when providers can demonstrate improved outcomes at a lower cost, and partner with payers to provide such care.

Collaborative care management is essential for reducing unnecessary hospital stays, and maximizing the time spent with patients in ambulatory settings. Integrating care through provider-directed, continuum-based clinical guidelines and pathways can further improve care by engaging the involvement of patients and families in collaborative relationships with providers and payers.

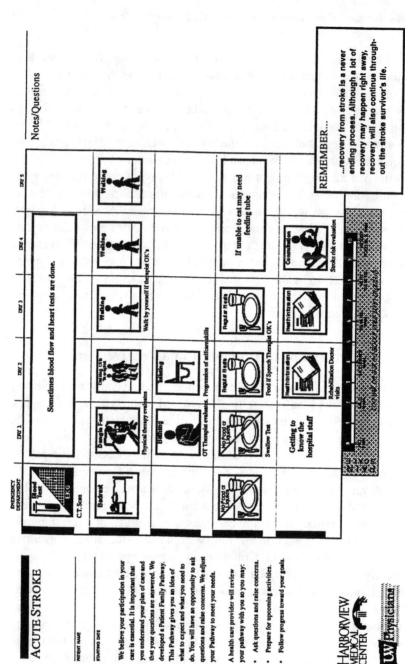

Figure 4.2 Patient pathway for acute stroke.

62

Chapter 5

Patients with Limited Health Literacy

Ruth M. Parker, Terry C. Davis, and Mark V. Williams

National surveys have documented that millions of Americans have inadequate literacy, and studies in the health care setting have confirmed that as patients, these same people struggle with health literacy demands. However, most practitioners are unaware of the magnitude of the problem, and physicians routinely take patients' ability to read and understand health-related materials for granted. Low-literate patients' ability to communicate with their health care providers and follow-up with self-care instructions is affected by limited health knowledge, poor understanding of basic health vocabulary, and difficulty assimilating new information and concepts (Doak et al., 1996). Simple instructions about how to take medications or prepare for diagnostic studies correctly, and directions for follow-up appointments, can be daunting to many low-literate patients. In this section, we overview literacy skills of Americans; health literacy and how it impacts patient-provider communication; how to identify patients with poor health literacy, and how to improve communication with low-literate patients. We conclude by looking at what health literacy means for patients in a market environment for health care delivery.

According to the National Adult Literacy Survey (NALS) (Kirsch, Jungeblut, Jenkins, & Kolstad, 1993) between 40 and 44 million Americans, or about one-fourth of the adult population, are functionally illiterate. This survey provided the most detailed portrait ever on the condition of literacy in our country. Twenty-two percent of the 13,600 adults who were surveyed for the NALS scored in the lowest of five skill levels. They struggle with tasks such as locating the expiration date on a driver's license or determining the location of a meeting on a form. Another 50 million Americans have only marginal literacy skills, as reflected by their scores in the second of five skill levels, which include locating an intersection on a street map and identifying and entering background information on a Social Security application. Overall, almost half of our adult population has basic deficiencies in reading, computational skills, or English. Importantly, among the 90 million Americans with limited literacy skills, only 15% were born outside the United States and only 5% reported having a learning disability. Inadequate literacy is especially common among the elderly, with nearly half scoring in the lowest skill level. This has important implications for health practitioners, since the elderly are most likely to have the greatest health-related reading needs due to the high prevalence of chronic diseases in this age group.

The National Literacy Act of 1991 defines literacy as "an individual's ability to read, write, and speak in English, and compute and solve problems at levels of proficiency necessary to function on the job and in society, to achieve one's goals, and develop one's knowledge and potential" (Public Law 102-73, 1991). Americans today reportedly have more education than at any time in our history; the average educational attainment of US adults is above the 12th grade level (Kirsch et al., 1993). However, the level of education does not necessarily translate into a corresponding reading level. Despite increasing overall education levels, average reading levels of US adults are between the 8th and 9th grade (Stedman & Kaestle, 1991). Reading, writing, and computational skills (i.e., literacy) better reflect functional ability than the level of educational attainment. Further, literacy skills are context- and setting-specific. Therefore, an individual may have adequate literacy skills in one content area, but inadequate skills in a different area or setting.

A growing body of literature is documenting the impact of limited literacy on the health care experience. With 40 million functionally illiterate American adults and 99 million Americans with chronic illnesses, there are countless instances every day where the health care system fails many of those most in need. In the largest study of health literacy, one third of English-speaking patients at two public hospitals were unable to read basic health materials (Williams, Parker, Baker, & Nurss, 1995). Forty-two percent of patients could not comprehend directions for taking medication on an empty stomach, 26% were unable to understand information on an appointment slip, 43% did not understand the rights and responsibilities section of a Medicaid application, and 60% did not understand a standard informed consent. A recent study of community-dwelling Medicare managed care patients in four cities enhanced the ability to generalize the earlier public hospital research on health literacy (Gazmararian, Baker, & Williams, 1999). In this study, 34% of English-speaking and 54% of Spanish-speaking Medicare patients had inadequate or marginal health literacy. Importantly, reading ability among the elderly declined very dramatically with age, even after adjusting for education level and cognitive impairment.

Impact of Health Literacy on Patient-Provider Communication

Patients' health literacy can be conceptualized as their currency for negotiating the health care system. The increasing importance of this currency is exemplified by the expansion of patient education requirements that has paralleled the exponential growth in medical technology. The following clinical example, initially cited in the American Medical Association's position paper on health literacy, demonstrates the relevance of this to practicing clinicians (Counsel on Scientific Affairs, 1999). Twenty-five years ago patients with newly diagnosed asthma were instructed to take theophylline, and encouraged to be diligent about compliance with follow-up appointments. Today, practitioners ask patients to monitor their disease with peak flow meters, select and correctly use the appropriate inhalers, sometimes augment therapy with tapering doses of oral steroids, and identify and avoid triggers that exacerbate their asthma. In addition, we expect them to use—but not overuse—the health care delivery system including the emergency department, their primary care physician, and subspecialists, and use these resources properly. The complexity of diagnosing and treating one of the most common chronic medical conditions challenges many physicians. Yet, we expect patients to acquire disease knowledge and complex self-management skills in busy practice settings that equate time with money.

When compounded by physicians' facile use of medical terms, patients' limited health vocabulary becomes a major source of miscommunication between them and their providers. Careful examination reveals that patients frequently feel that their physicians do not adequately explain illnesses or treatment plans in understandable terms (Mayeaux et al., 1996). Many busy practitioners probably are aware that some misunderstanding exists between them and their patients, but they hope that easily accessible educational brochures will help patients clarify their understanding and answer any remaining questions. Unfortunately, there is a growing disparity between patients' reading abilities and their health literacy needs (Counsel on Scientific Affairs, 1999). Numerous studies now document that many health materials, including patient education brochures, discharge instruction sheets, contraception instructions, and informed consent documents, often are written at levels that far exceed patients' reading abilities.

Patients with low literacy and poor knowledge of health vocabulary and concepts obtain less information from health education materials (Doak et al., 1996). They may be overwhelmed with information, yet too uncomfortable to ask questions. Providers often give too much background material, rather than information that helps patients solve their problems. This may result in poor adherence. Patients with poor health literacy often take the wrong doses of medications or take their medications at the wrong frequency, and they may not be aware of important treatment side effects or the need for follow-up testing (Baker, Parker, & Williams, 1996). They may interpret instructions literally, misunderstand the context, or be unable to make inferences from factual data (Davis, Williams, Branch, & Green, 1999). Patients with inadequate health literacy who have chronic diseases such as hypertension, diabetes, or asthma know less about their diseases than those whose literacy skills are adequate (Williams et al., 1998; Williams, Baker, Honig, et al., 1998). Therefore providers should not assume routinely that patients correctly understand their diagnoses and treatment plans.

Health care is becoming increasingly complex and more reliant on written materials for patient education (Davis et al., 1999). Many managed care organizations use regular newsletters to communicate with patients about self-management issues of their chronic diseases. Poor health literacy also may be a barrier to preventive health measures. Many public health messages and education materials about recommended disease prevention and screening are inaccessible to those with low literacy. For example, those with low literacy may not read and understand messages about the value of mammography or flu shots that may be found in magazines, on billboards, or on clinic posters.

Identifying Patients with Poor Health Literacy

People with limited literacy may not recognize or admit their reading difficulty; remarkably, two-thirds of those who tested in the lowest skill level of NALS describe themselves as being able to read "well" or "very well." In a study of shame and health literacy, shame was common among patients with low literacy who acknowledged they had trouble reading (Parikh et al., 1996). Shame is a deeply harbored emotion that probably plays an important role in understanding how patients with low literacy feel. Illiteracy carries a stigma and creates feelings of inadequacy and poor self-esteem which in our society probably is one of the main reasons many individuals hide their inability to read. When asked to read in front of their physician, patients with low literacy might hide their difficulty by saying, "I forgot my reading glasses," "I'd like to discuss this with my family first; may I take the instructions home?" or "I don't need to read this through now; I'll read it when I get home." Patients with low literacy vary greatly (Weiss & Coyne, 1997) and providers should not assume they can readily identify which patients have poor health literacy.

Actual assessment of patients' reading skills can help health care providers find more effective ways to communicate with their patients (Davis et al., 1999). By testing a sample of patients in a clinic or hospital setting, providers can better select and develop educational interventions that are appropriate for the health literacy level of their target population.

There are tests available for assessing patients' literacy in the office setting. The Rapid Estimate of Adult Literacy in Medicine (REALM) (Davis, Long, & Jackson, 1993) is a word recognition test which assesses patients' ability to read from a list of progressively more difficult words until they encounter words they cannot pronounce correctly. The REALM was developed for use in the clinical setting; it is simple to use and score and can be completed in 5 minutes or less. However, it is not valid in Spanish and does not assess patients' numeracy, or quantitative literacy.

The Test of Functional Health Literacy in Adults (TOFHLA) was developed to test patients' ability to read passages and phrases using real materials from the health care setting (Parker, Baker, Williams, & Nurss, 1995). The TOFHLA was the first available tool for measuring functional health literacy, or patients' ability to perform health-related tasks that require reading and computational skills. Reading passages on the TOFHLA were selected from instructions for preparation for an upper gastrointestinal series, the patient rights and responsibilities sections of a Medicaid application form, and a standard hospital informed consent form. The numeracy items test patients' ability to comprehend directions for taking medicines, monitoring blood glucose, keeping clinic appointments, and obtaining financial assistance. Although the TOFHLA is a valid and reliable tool, it takes up to 22 minutes to administer. To overcome this, the short TOFHLA (S-TOFHLA) was developed (Baker et al., in press). Maximum time for administration was reduced to 12 minutes, and the S-TOFHLA is a practical measure of functional health literacy which has good reliability and validity.

There is no "gold standard" for measuring health literacy (Baker et al., in press). Patients who completed 8 or fewer years of school are very likely to have inadequate health literacy, and those who completed education beyond high school are likely to have adequate functional health literacy. However, the NALS found that 16% to 20% of adults with high school diplomas scored in the lowest proficiency level. Without formal testing, it is difficult to identify those with health literacy problems among the large proportion of patients who completed 9–12 years of school. The S-TOFHLA measures patients' ability to read and understand actual health texts, while the REALM measures their ability to pronounce words in isolation. The TOFHLA has been shown to independently predict patients' knowledge of chronic disease and self-management skills, health status, and use of health care services. Patients' REALM scores have been associated with women's knowledge and attitudes about mammography. Further studies are needed to determine relative advantages and disadvantages of the S-TOFHLA and REALM.

Recognizing reading difficulties does not always require testing with a standardized instrument. One author (R. Parker) identifies patients with reading problems by asking them to read the label on a pill bottle which she keeps in her coat pocket. Practitioners also may be suspicious when patients fill out intake forms incorrectly or return survey risk forms with all items checked. The most important point is that practitioners should not routinely assume that all patients have adequate health literacy.

Improving Communication with Low-Literate Patients

Providers who discover that a substantial portion of their patients have health literacy problems will need to carefully evaluate and probably revise the overall educational approach used in their clinical setting (Davis et al., 1999). Clinic staff need to be sensitized to how anxious and ashamed some patients are about being expected to correctly read and complete intake forms and informed consent documents, or follow complex instructions for diagnostic studies. Instituting a system where help is routinely offered in completing important documents, and where surrogate readers for patients with limited health literacy are included when important health education is communicated, can help to circumvent some of the problems.

Clinicians also should consider using nonwritten materials to communicate information to patients with limited health literacy (Weiss & Coyne, 1997). Even patients who read well often prefer nonwritten materials, including straightforward picture books, videotapes, audiotapes, or multimedia presentations. When written materials are crucial, they should be prepared at the fifth-grade level or lower. Health educators stress that people of all literacy levels prefer materials that are simple and easy to understand (Doak et al., 1996). Many standard patient education materials are written at a high school or college level, and are thus inaccessible to many patients.

During clinical encounters, health care providers need to make their communication "fit" their patients' actual health literacy. A few simple techniques include slowing down, using simple language, and including a family member in discussions. Clinicians and health educators often inadvertently hinder communication by providing complex background information that has little to do with what patients need to know to care for themselves. Instead, clinicians need to do more to ensure patient understanding. Health educators have advocated a "teach back" or "show me" approach (Doak et al., 1996). Providers demonstrate a desired skill (e.g., checking a blood glucose level or using an inhaler) to patients, rather than asking patients to read about the skill. They then ask them to demonstrate the skill to assure they have correct understanding. Practitioners can make patients feel more comfortable about being "tested" by asking the patient to teach back to them what they just explained so they can judge their own abilities as teachers. For example, "Could you now tell me or show me what I just went over with you? I need to see how well I did explaining this to you. This is important so we both feel like you will know how to take care of yourself at home."

Some patients with health literacy problems may use "surrogate" readers to help them understand what they need to do to take care of their medical problems. Surrogates may include family members, close friends, or sometimes a neighbor. Often these important caretakers are not present at the time that the provider gives critical health education about further diagnostic studies, treatment options or plans, or self-care instructions. "Surrogate readers" for patients with health literacy difficulties should be included in conversations about health education and instructions for self-care. To ensure the provider that the surrogate has adequate comprehension of instructions, they need to be involved in the "teach back" as well.

Providing high-quality care to patients with health literacy problems requires spending time on patient education. The "information-giving" time that patients so value is shrinking (Davidoff, 1997) in practice settings that increasingly seem to equate time with money. The next section examines more closely the meaning of health literacy for patients and their providers in such an environment.

Health Literacy and the "Market" for Health Care

Access to medical services and delivery of health care frequently are described in the context of "the market." Traditionally recognized characteristics of a market include the notion of a sovereign consumer. This implies that an individual who chooses to buy a good or service is expressing a self-interest and is optimally informed about the full range of available products, including their quality, prices, and likely consequences. What does health literacy have to do with consumers of health and health care in a market environment?

This question can be explored by looking at health care choices currently being formulated for Medicare patients in our country. Medicare+Choice (Medicare Part C) was created by the 1997 Balanced Budget Act to increase the number of seniors who get health care from managed care rather than traditional fee-for-service Medicare. Initial plans for introducing Medicare+Choice are as follows. Every beneficiary in five states receives a handbook describing the specific health plans available in each region. This includes a worksheet to help them select a different plan than the one they already have. The 33.5 million beneficiaries in the other 45 states receive a bulletin introducing them to the idea of new health plan choices. The bulletin also will assure them that if they are happy with the way they receive health care now, they do not need to take any action. Beneficiaries are advised to consult new comparison charts being put together by the Health Care Financing Organization (HCFA). One such chart will list all health plans by zip code on the Internet (www.Medicare.gov) and include information on the copayments, deductibles, and basic benefits they offer. Over the years, HCFA will collect and post plan-specific quality measures, including information on how plans scored on Health Plan Employer Data and Information Set (HEDIS) standardized performance measures. The goal is to enable beneficiaries to compare health plans and choose one based not only on cost but also on how well it provides certain services.

A recent study of more than 3,000 Prudential Medicare beneficiaries in four cities found that 34% of English speaking patients and 54% of Spanish-speaking patients had inadequate or marginal health literacy (Gazmararian et al., 1999). These patients struggle to read their pill bottles and appointment slips. How can they function as informed sovereign consumers in a health care market?

Managed care settings offer new challenges and opportunities for addressing patients' health literacy. Studies of patients' health literacy abilities and needs within individual plans can help the plans design specific interventions, targeted to subgroups of their high-risk enrollees (e.g., older patients; those with less education) (Gazmararian et al., 1999). Encouraging and providing the best possible care for our patients requires real communication, not just "words." Patients, their families, doctors and other providers, and health care delivery organizations must truly partner to address the pressing health literacy needs of our patients.

Chapter 6

Multiculturalism: Patient and Provider Diversity

Esther Chachkes

In recent decades, the United States has become more ethnically and culturally diverse (McLaughlin & Braun, 1998). Currently, more than 31 million people in the United States do not speak English as their first language (U.S. Bureau of the Census, 1993). Each ethnic group brings its own perspectives and values to the health care arena, and many of their health care beliefs and health practices differ from those of the mainstream American health care culture. Nonetheless, the implicit, if not explicit, expectation of many health care providers too often has been that patients will conform to mainstream values. Such expectations frequently have created barriers to care which have been complicated by differences in language and education between patient and health care provider when they come from different backgrounds. Valuing multiculturalism is a recent paradigm shift, but it has resulted in an increasing emphasis on cross-cultural understanding on the part of health care providers (Irish, Lundquist, & Nelsen, 1993). Greater awareness of diversity and attention to the needs of special populations, and training to further these ends, is now a mandate of the Joint Commission for the Accreditation of Hospitals (JCAHO) (JCAHO, 1993).

Culture is "the integrated pattern of human behavior that includes thoughts, communications, actions, customs, beliefs, values, and institutions of a racial, ethnic, religious or social group" (Cross, Bazron, Dennis, & Issacs, 1989, p. 3). Health care professionals have not always been aware of their own cultural perspectives, how pervasively different another individual's culture may be, and how subtly such cultural differences may manifest themselves. Cultural differences form the entire context in which a person's knowledge, attitudes, understanding, and behavior are demonstrated. To be effective in our roles as healers, health care providers must be aware of and sensitive to differences in the health knowledge, attitudes, beliefs, and practices of individuals and families whose cultural frameworks and perspectives differ from ours. Unless we can achieve a common ground, access barriers may be strengthened rather than minimized, resulting in decreased utilization of services, poor adherence to treatment regimens, and possibly, a higher incidence of poor outcomes.

The mandate for cultural competence grows stronger as we strive to reduce the disparities in health care delivery. The challenge is to integrate knowledge and understanding of cultural issues and the social conditions in which ethnic minorities live into health care service delivery so we can improve the health status of these populations. The aim of this chapter is to provide busy clinicians with a brief background on cultural diversity and cultural competence and a few helpful tools that will help them to practice more effectively when dealing with patients whose backgrounds are significantly different from their own.

Cultural Diversity

Cultural differences affect patients' attitudes about medical care and their ability to understand, manage, and cope with the course of an illness, the meaning of a diagnosis, and the consequences of medical treatment. Patients and their caregivers bring culture-specific ideas and values related to concepts of health and illness, reporting of symptoms, expectations for how health care will be delivered, and beliefs concerning medication and treatments to the health care encounter. In addition, culture-specific values influence patient roles and expectations, how much information about illness and treatment is desired, how death and dying will be managed, bereavement patterns, gender and family roles, and processes for decision-making.

Cross-cultural variations also exist within cultures. Discussions about culture are generalizations; individual behaviors are influenced by a variety of issues, including personality, individual experiences, social class, educational levels, and religious influences. Geographic locations within a country can also create variations in cultural themes. Chow (1996) discusses how community centers in Chinatowns across America must learn about the different needs of immigrants from Fuzhou, Shanghai, Beijing, and Taiwan contrasted with those previous immigrants who came primarily from Taisan and Canton.

The degree of cultural assimilation and knowledge of English also influence how individuals adapt to a new culture and their ability to move between cultures with ease. An article in Case Management Advisor lists six points in a continuum of assimilation patterns ranging from traditional to bicultural: individuals totally committed to their original culture; acculturated individuals who value open communication and ideas from both cultures; culturally assimilated persons who adopt the new culture; individuals who function in both cultures (cultural pluralism); culturally immersed persons who adopt the new culture, but place more value on the original culture; and bicultural individuals who move between both cultures easily. Within each family, different members may be at different points of the continuum, depending on migration status. It is important to understand the degree of assimilation of all family members.

With shorter lengths of stay and a shift to outpatient care, including care in the home, the ability to provide appropriate care to a culturally diverse population necessitates an understanding of how these cultural influences impact on the ways in which people use health care and are able to manage the expectations of mainstream American medical care. Patients and caregivers must be prepared to manage care without readily available professional expertise. The challenge of managing many of the newer and more complex treatments is difficult for the most competent and resourceful patients. For those who speak a language other than English, or whose culture has not prepared them for the reality of such health care technologies, it is much greater, and the potential for error is much higher. Patient involvement, understanding, and preparation is necessary in order to insure that distribution of resources will not be limited because of educational needs.

Cultural Variations in Health Care Beliefs

All cultures have systems of health beliefs to explain the causality of illness, how it can be cured or treated, and who should be involved in the process. Cultural perspectives determine which symptoms are viewed as health-related and therefore to be reported, whether they are to be treated, and how. Cultural views of illness also determine the medicinal preparations and environmental conditions that are deemed necessary for treatment, and they identify the persons who are able to treat and cure.

Kavanagh and Kennedy (1992) relate the belief in the etiology of illness to the therapies promoted for its treatment. For example, more scientific societies place etiology in natural phenomena. Treatments are then based on combating microorganisms or environmental or emotional disturbances. When illness is believed to be the result of supernatural phenomena, prayer or other interventions that can counter the presumed disfavor of powerful forces will be invoked. If illness is viewed as the result of poor social interactions or social problems, treatments aimed at altering social structures or social arrangements are preferred.

Building upon Arthur Kleinman's seminal work (Kleinman, Eisenberg, & Good, 1978) on the development of a health explanatory belief model, Susan Hopper (1993) has developed a list of questions that can assist providers in gaining a better understanding of a patient's perspective on their health problems. These questions include:

> What do you think is wrong with you?
> How serious do you think your problem is?
> What do you think caused this problem?
> Why do you think this problem has happened to you now?
> What are some of the things you do to help with this problem?
> What are some of the things that you have always done to keep yourself healthy and strong?
> How likely is it that the treatment that you are now getting will help your condition?
> (If taking medicines) How does this medicine work?
> How likely is it that you will be able to follow the advice you have been given about how to take care of yourself and this problem?
> Have you experienced any problems as a result of the advice or treatments that you have received?
> Compared to others whom you know, are you doing better than average?
> What are some of the changes in your life as a result of having this problem?
> Which of the following best describes your feelings about your health:
> a) Most of what happens to your health is a matter of chance
> b) There are many things that you can do to improve your health.

The types of questions asked can vary. The critical aspects of the assessment are that the questions elicit sufficient information, that they are asked in a nonjudgmental manner, and that advice is not offered.

Views toward illness reflect the range of cultural responses. The following discussion of particular cultural perspectives is offered as an illustration of the many ways in which cultural perspectives affect individual behavior.

Most cultures have a proscribed way of viewing the etiology of mental illness. Among Chinese patients, somatic complaints are more easily tolerated than psychological ones because all individual behaviors reflect upon the family. Family harmony is a significant cultural value, mental illness may suggest a lack of self-constraint and self-control, attributes that can evoke considerable shame and guilt. Traditional Chinese values emphasize the importance of individual will-power and lack of morbid thinking as contributing to sound mental health (Dillard, 1983). As a result, many Chinese patients will be reluctant to discuss symptoms of mental illness, and they may not view these as indicative of psychological illness. In Hindu and Moslem cultures, where individuals in the family with emotional illness or mental retardation may reduce chances of marriage for siblings, there may be a reluctance to acknowledge emotional illness.

Mental problems often are explained by mystical beliefs. In Vietnamese culture, health is viewed as the result of a harmonious balance between the two poles of hot and cold that govern bodily functions. Maintaining the equilibrium of hot and cold is essential, and medicines can assist in this. Winds also determine physical and mental well-being—"phong" or wind can enter the body and cause distress. Vietnamese believe that psychological problems are the result of supernatural forces whose anger will strike an individual who has not adhered to appropriate religious standards. Mental illness is highly stigmatized; it is a cause for family shame. The family is of critical importance in Vietnamese culture and family structure is hierarchical. The extended family system, past and present, influences identity. Individual identity is linked to a line of ancestors (Dillard, 1983). Mental illness suggests a failure of the individual, ridicules the line of ancestors, and causes a "loss of face" within the community. This poses a reluctance to accept Western mental health counseling which involves disclosure of the problem.

For the Amish, mental illness may be viewed as an inability to find satisfaction with work or marriage. Healing is sought through work rather than focusing on problems (Randall-Davis, 1989). Family and community are involved as important members of the patient's social support system, and advice will be sought from respected members of the community. The family, with several generations living together in the same household, is the primary support system, and is expected to aid in times of crisis and stress (Wittmer, 1995). The role of professionals generally is not a significant one.

Different cultural groups also bring attitudes about the health care system based on their prior experiences. For example, Russian immigrants to the United States view American medical care with great distrust because relationships with medical practitioners in the former Soviet Union were authoritarian and free exchange of information and open discussion did not often occur. Diagnoses were not disclosed, prognosis was not discussed, and reasons for surgery were not shared. As a result, Russian patients often find it difficult to communicate with a physician and to talk openly about medical concerns. They expect a paternalistic approach, equating it with competency. American insistence on self-management and patient involvement in decision-making may seem contradictory to their traditional understanding of patient roles and behavior (Brod & Heurtin-Roberts, 1992). Further, given their previous experience with the dangers of psychiatric hospitalizations, there is a reluctance to share information about personal matters. Manipulation of the authority figure is considered a more effective coping mechanism.

Fatalistic views of illness also influence management. For example, in Hispanic cultures, illness is viewed as "God's will" or divine punishment. It also may be seen as resulting from suffering that is intrinsic to the human condition (Chachkes & Jennings, 1994). To engender trust, health care providers must have strong listening skills and respect for bicultural differences, and develop supportive relationships. Through close relationships, Hispanic patients can be encouraged to comply with medical regimes.

The Amish believe that the human body is divinely created and will be healed by God. A healthy person is one who eats well, works hard, and therefore looks well. Although medical interventions are accepted, their power to heal is secondary. Amish society does not prohibit using medical services, but there is a well-developed folk healing system which uses home remedies and folk healers who provide "sympathy healing." The "pow-wow" is an example of community involvement used to promote cure (Randall-Davis, 1989). Medical interventions with the Amish will be more effective if they include an understanding of such cultural values as humility, keeping social distance from nonAmish, maintaining a sober and quiet demeanor in public, and using at least three Amish adults for advice with problem-solving and decision-making (Wittmer, 1995).

Haitians believe that many illnesses are related to supernatural causes. Voodoo is the preferred method to rid the person of evil spirits. If illness is caused by natural reasons, it is considered a result of blood irregularities. The interventions of voodoo priests and family to help the individual may be very productive. However, this is often difficult for Western practitioners to accept (Randall-Davis, 1989).

Gender roles can have an impact on how care is sought and received. In most Asian societies, women are often subordinate and are expected to be obedient, unassuming, yielding, timid, respectful, reticent, and unselfish (Mo, 1992). This role behavior affects an Asian woman's relationship to health care providers. Amish society is patriarchal, and women are expected to be submissive.

In Hispanic cultures, men are expected to be rebellious, while women are to be modest, submissive, and obedient. Men are expected to protect women (*machismo*) and to provide for their care. Treatment options may be discussed and decided upon after conferring with influential members of the extended family or community, and husbands may be the ultimate decision-makers about health practices. This has been a particular issue in the use of condoms for HIV prevention. Consequently, educational interventions must consider the limited ability of women to influence safer sexual practices.

Promptness may be critical in some cultures, while others may not emphasize strict adherence to time schedules and view time more flexibly. Anglo-Americans tend to be clock-watchers, while Hispanics may show up late for appointments without showing concern; reciprocally, however, Hispanics may then be more comfortable waiting their turn than will members of other cultures. Attitudes about time are culturally linked. In today's busy managed care system, where schedules, appointments, and medication times are very important to the delivery of health care, time considerations must be understood.

Cross-Cultural Communication

Cross-cultural understanding is an interactive process which affects health care providers as well as patients and families. When a patient speaks a different language, or is part of a culture in which current treatments and the nature of the diagnosis are not discussed, the entire teaching process must be tailored to take into account cultural factors that may impede learning. Language skills, intelligence, comfort in asking questions, dealing with authority, motivation, and readiness to listen to information that may be new or anxiety-provoking also must be taken into account. Sometimes patients must be encouraged to learn new ways of approaching care and to accept necessary changes.

The Patient's Bill of Rights and the Patient Self-Determination Act are based on American values for the individual's rights to self-determination in health care decision making. This has become imbedded in current American health care policy. When cultures value collective decision making over individual preferences, requirements for informed consent and advance directives can be problematic. The health care provider must be the arbitrator between the patient/family and the health care system—helping those from other cultures understand the legal aspects of these policies, but modifying them to be more culturally acceptable. In collectivist societies, families and groups make decisions. For example, in the case of many Chinese and Japanese patients, the oldest son is assigned decision-making authority. Because concerns about death and dying are not easily expressed verbally, in Chinese culture, it would be improper for an elder son to discuss this with his parents. This becomes an important issue when advance directives or do-not-resuscitate orders must be discussed. In Pacific Island families, conversely, a variety of family members are assigned caregiving duties, and all family members are expected to receive the same level of detail about the patient's diagnosis, prognosis, and treatment options (McLaughlin & Braun).

The issue of folk medicine, healers, and alternative therapies and therapists is a complex one. When these therapies are not likely to be harmful, integrating indigenous practices and practitioners into care can encourage trust and foster communication. However, it may be necessary to respectfully disagree when these practices are considered dangerous or at serious variance with accepted medical practice.

Health care providers must also learn about culturally correct patterns of communication and differences in verbal expressiveness and affective behaviors. Some cultures (e.g., Latino/Latina) prefer highly expressive modes of communication while others (e.g., Asians) value more subdued modes. The acceptability of talking to professionals can also vary between cultural groups. For Asians, polite, restrained behavior is the norm; for Hispanics, more emotive expressions are acceptable. Anglo-Americans value directness and open communication.

Nonverbal communication styles can be equally important. For example, Orthodox Jewish men will not shake hands with women. Asian women may not shake hands with each other or with men. In certain Asian groups, touching the head, eye-to-eye contact, waving arms with palms upward, and pointing at things with one's toe are all actions considered to be rude.

Some cultures value nonverbal approaches to communication more than verbal approaches, and verbal answers may be short and offered only when requested, as in Native American cultures (Kavanagh & Kennedy, 1992). Long periods of silence are acceptable.

In Hispanic cultures, establishing a personal relationship (*personalismo*) is important and is seen as a sign of respect. A compliment for the health care provider is to be described as a "good friend" or "like a cousin" (Chachkes & Jennings, 1994). For the Amish, polite listening to advice is acceptable, but the advice will not be acted upon until it is discussed with members of the community.

People take great pride in their culture and the nationalism that often marks their identification with their country of origin. Effective communication respects this and is dependent upon an understanding of the cultural framework that determines an individual's health-related behavior. In addition, cross-cultural assessments must include an understanding of English proficiency and literacy of both English and the native language; health beliefs, gender-related issues, age, education, degree of acculturation, and social class all influence the relationship between provider and patient. It is also imperative that providers understand the great pride newcomers take in their culture and the nationalism that often marks their identification in this country. Many recent immigrants to the US have come here as refugees and experienced multiple traumas such as war, famine, or torture. If possible, a full migration history should be obtained; where this is not possible, learning as much as possible about what has happened in the past, and acknowledging the traumatic experiences of these individuals can help to bond providers and patients.

Cultural Assessments

Cultural competence requires that a practitioner know how to gain information about patients' health care beliefs and practices. This knowledge forms the basis for the development of a treatment and care plan that is culturally appropriate and will be acceptable to the patient. In order to gain knowledge, however, practitioners must be culturally sensitive and aware and have good communication skills.

Communication is a complex process. It involves sophisticated listening skills, an ability to analyze situations from the perspective of diversity, and a respect for differences. Kavanagh and Kennedy (1992) believe that communication is the first challenge in working with diversity, and that awareness, sensitivity, and knowledge alone cannot successfully encourage meaningful cross-cultural interventions. They cite several areas for cross-cultural communication skills: ability to articulate and present an issue from the perspective of another culture; recognizing and reducing defensiveness, and acceptance of interactive mistakes (Kavanagh & Kennedy, 1992). A skilled communicator can understand communication patterns that conflict with mainstream American patterns, including verbal and nonverbal responses, and can modify interactions accordingly. Social status and hierarchical factors also influence communication. This is important for health care providers to keep in mind, as most patients view medical personnel as holding higher rank. Kavanagh and Kennedy list 20 goals to facilitate communication among members of diverse groups. They include:

Promote a feeling of acceptance;
Strive to gain another's trust;
Understand the relationships with authority;
Avoid assumptions about people—let them tell you instead;
Show respect;
Know about traditional health care beliefs and practices, including folk remedies; and
Make the setting comfortable and learn to appreciate the richness of diversity.

Dillard (1983) describes the basic communication skills as understanding cultural patterns of appropriate eye contact, body language and proximity preferences, tone of voice and speech rate and appropriateness of certain subjects for discussion. In some cultures, direct eye contact is viewed as staring, while in others too-frequent breaks in eye contact may be interpreted as a lack of concern. Body language varies greatly, and is an important aspect of communication. All cultures have a preference for comfortable physical distance and personal space requirements. Initiating a discussion about subjects that may be unacceptable can be very difficult. Awareness of whether the subject is taboo or not can help the health care provider introduce the subject in a more culturally sensitive manner.

Vace, DeVaney, and Wittmar (1995) cite the importance of awareness of one's own culture, which facilitates learning about another culture. Understanding one's own cultural roots and its biases, stereotypes, and values enables one to learn about other groups. Basic values can differ from culture to culture and influence decision making and the acceptance of medical care. For example, Americans tend to value personal growth and changes; other cultures may see conformity as a higher goal. Americans believe in individual control, rather than control by external forces. Different values are placed on the importance of professional help and the trustworthiness of professionals. There also are differences regarding when open discussions of problems can be held, and with whom (Vace, DeVaney, & Wittmar, 1995). Health care providers are not value-neutral. Therefore, we must be aware of our own cultural backgrounds and values. Without this self-awareness, our risk of coercing patients is higher.

McLaughlin and Braun (1998) recommend the following strategies for helping professionals who work in cross-cultural settings:

1. Learn about the cultural traditions of the groups with which you are working.

2. Pay close attention to body language, lack of response, or feelings of tension that may signify that the patient or family is in conflict but are perhaps hesitant to tell you.

3. Ask the patient and family open-ended questions to elicit more information about their assumptions and expectations.

4. Remain non-judgmental when provided with information that reflects values that differ from your own.

5. Follow the advice given to you by your clients about appropriate ways to facilitate communication within families and between families and other health care providers.

These authors conclude that the primary aid in cross-cultural communication is sensitivity and awareness, and they encourage education and training to promote understanding and appreciation of diverse cultures (McLaughlin & Braun, 1998).

Summary

Without total immersion, it is nearly impossible to become totally knowledgeable about another culture. However, it is possible to achieve cultural competence. Several mnemonics can be useful for cross-cultural communication. The first is to think ETHNIC (Table 6.1). When dealing with psychosocial issues, BATHE (Table 6.2), should be helpful. While this chapter has not discussed the myriad of issues relating to the use of medical interpreters, TRANSLATE (Table 6.3) summarizes them well and provides useful advice. Finally, LEARN (Table 6.4) summarizes the advice we have provided.

Respecting cultural pluralism necessitates an interactive process, with the health care provider learning from the patient and family about their knowledge, attitudes, beliefs, and practices, while also teaching the patient and family about the dominant American health care culture. The result will be a more culturally competent approach that promotes greater access to health care and more effective utilization of health services.

Table 6.1   ETHNIC—A Framework for Culturally Competent Clinical Practice

Explanation—"Why do you think you have these symptoms? What do your friends, family and others say about them? Do you know anyone else who has had or who has this kind of problem?"

Treatment—"Do you take any medications, home remedies or other treatments for this illness or to stay healthy? What kind of treatment are you seeking from me?"

Healers—"Have you sought advice from family, friends, alternative/folk healers or other non-physicians?"

Negotiate—Negotiate *mutually acceptable* treatment options that incorporate your patient's beliefs without contradicting yours. Ask your patient the most important results he or she hopes to achieve from the intervention.

Intervention—Determine the intervention with your patient. Recognize that it may include incorporation of alternative treatments, spirituality, healers and other cultural practices (e.g., foods eaten or avoided in general and when sick).

Collaborate—Collaborate with the patient, family, health team members, healers and community resources.

Table 6.2   BATHE—A Useful Mnemonic for Eliciting
the Psychosocial Context

Background—A simple question such as "What is going on in your life?" elicits the context of the patient's visit.

Affect—Asking, "How do you feel about what is going on?" or "What is your mood?" allows the patient to report and label the current feeling state.

Trouble—"What about the situation troubles you the most?" helps the physician and patient focus, and may bring out the symbolic significance of the illness or event.

Handling—"How are you handling that?" gives an assessment of functioning and provides direction for an intervention.

Empathy—"That must be very difficult for you" legitimizes the patient's feelings and provides psychological support (Stuart & Lieberman, 1993).

Table 6.3   TRANSLATE—A Mnemonic for Working With
Medical Interpreters

Trust—How will trust be developed in the patient-clinician-interpreter triadic relationship? In relationships with the patient's family and other health care professionals?

Roles—What role(s) will the interpreter play in the clinical care process (e.g., language translator, culture broker/informant, culture broker/interpreter of biomedical culture, advocate)?

Advocacy—How will advocacy and support for patient- and family-centered care occur? How will power and loyalty issues be handled?

Nonjudgmental attitude—How can a nonjudgmental attitude be maintained during health care encounters? How will personal beliefs, values, opinions, biases, and stereotypes be dealt with?

Setting—Where and how will medical interpretation occur during health care encounters (e.g., use of salaried interpreters, volunteers, AT&T Language Line)?

Language—What methods of communication will be employed? How will linguistic appropriateness and competence be stressed?

Accuracy—How will knowledge and information be exchanged in an accurate, thorough, and complete manner during health care encounters?

Time—How will time be managed appropriately during health care encounters?

Ethical Issues—How will potential ethical conflicts be handled during health care encounters? How will confidentiality of clinical information be maintained?

From "Communication Through Interpreters in Healthcare: Ethical Dilemmas Arising from Differences in Class, Culture, Language, and Power," by J. M. Kaufert and R. W. Putsch, 1977, *Journal of Clinical Ethics*, 8(1). Adapted with permission.

Table 6.4   LEARN—A Teaching Framework for Cross Cultural Health Care

Listen with sympathy and understanding to the patient's perception of the problem.

Explain your perception of the problem.

Acknowledge and discuss the differences and similarities.

Recommend treatment.

Negotiate agreement.

Note: From "A Teaching Framework for Cross-Cultural Health Care," by E. A. Berlin and W. C. Fowkes Jr., 1983, *Western Journal of Medicine 139*. Reprinted with permission.

PART II

Working with Specific Patient Populations

Chapter 7

Health Promotion and Disease Prevention

Elizabeth J. Kramer

More than 80% of our current illness burden is a result of chronic diseases occurring in people between the ages of 55 and their deaths (Fries et al., 1998). Approximately 70% of the burden of illness and its associated costs is preventable. A study which reclassified causes of death found that eight of the nine leading causes of death were preventable. In rank order from highest to lowest they are: cigarette smoking, lack of exercise, suboptimal diet, low birth weight, injury resulting from failure to use seat belts or safety helmets, trauma associated with alcohol or other substance abuse, and sexually transmitted diseases (Fries et al., 1998).

In large part, good health is a function of individual assumption of responsibility for health. Success in this effort requires individuals to possess personal self-efficacy, which can be defined as the belief that one may be able to affect health by personal behavior. Self-efficacy is an essential prerequisite for subsequent changes in health risk behavior. A growing body of evidence suggests that people who are confident that they can affect their health, are more likely to modify their behavior than those who lack such confidence. This "perceived self-efficacy" can be enhanced through skills mastery, modeling, reinterpreting the meaning of symptoms, and persuasion.

Many thanks to Richard Levy and Michael Sofia for their contributions to the section on medication teaching.

In a 1994 survey of practicing primary care physicians in Massachusetts, 89% said that it was "definitely" their responsibility to educate patients about health-related risk factors, and the majority reported feeling "very prepared" to counsel patients about smoking, alcohol use, and exercise. However fewer than half felt "very prepared" to counsel patients about diet, stress, depression, or illicit drug use (Wechsler, Levine, & Idelson, 1996).

Definitions

Health promotion is "any combination of educational, organizational, economic and environmental supports for behavior and conditions of living conducive to health" (Green, 1992, p. 793). In an expanded definition, health promotion includes "all activities that educate, guide, and motivate the individual to take personal actions which improve the likelihood of sustained good health and increase the appropriateness of requested services" (Fries et al., 1998, pp. 76–77).

Health promotion is the first step in disease prevention. It focuses on the modification of personal health behaviors to reduce the risk of disease and injury. Health promotion is the common vector of public health and clinical medicine. It is primarily a public health function which is delivered through multiple media including but not necessarily limited to billboard, newspaper, and magazine advertising, and articles, public service announcements, and educational programs on television and radio, as well as educational materials produced by various voluntary health agencies, such as the American Heart Association and the American Diabetes Association, that are targeted to the avoidance of unhealthy habits (e.g., smoking and substance abuse) and the development and implementation of good habits (e.g., diet and exercise and regular seat belt usage). Education in primary prevention and health promotion is targeted to modification of lifestyle issues. Clinical activities tend to focus on activities such as immunizations and screening for infectious and chronic diseases.

Disease prevention has three levels: primary, secondary, and tertiary. Primary prevention involves the prevention of disease before it begins; secondary prevention identifies and treats asymptomatic persons who already have developed risk factors or preclinical disease, but in whom the disease itself has not become clinically apparent; and the aim of tertiary prevention is to prevent or slow deterioration resulting from chronic disease.

Screening

Screening for diseases that either can be prevented in their entirety, or for which early intervention will prolong both length and quality of life, and periodic, targeted medical examinations are opportune times for teaching and reinforcing self care. The United States Preventive Services Task Force has recommended age-specific screening procedures for the general population and procedures for those in each age group who are at risk for specific diseases. These recommendations for adolescents and adults are shown in Tables 7.1 through 7.4.

In customizing the recommendations to their practices or individual patients, providers should consider each patient's age, medical, and social history. For example, seat belt usage, the dangers of drinking and driving, the hazards of drug abuse, and sexually transmitted disease prevention should be emphasized with adolescents and young adults. Where appropriate, the hazards of handgun usage should be added to this list. Prevention of heart disease, cancer, and problem drinking should be emphasized in young and middle-aged adults. In the case of older patients, emphasis is placed on the same diseases as middle age, but should be supplemented by attention to sensory impairments, disturbances of gait, and depression.

Patient Education

Education in primary prevention and health promotion is targeted to modification of lifestyle issues. Health care providers, especially primary care practitioners, have a unique opportunity to influence behavioral risk factors, since the motivation to seek health care already has delineated a self-selected population who are receptive to receiving educational and therapeutic interventions. Further, the clinical setting is a good place to offer positive reinforcements such as initial encouragement to modify a behavior, a medical rationale to help patients perceive the benefits of behavioral change, the credibility of medical expertise and familiarity with individual patients' medical histories, suggestions for strategies of behavioral change that fit their medical, social, and economic circumstances, an authoritative referral for outside help, and periodic support of their progress during subsequent medical encounters. Social support can be stimulated by asking family members to come to visits with patients or by treating the family as a unit (Green, 1992).

Table 7.1   Screening Recommendations for People Ages 11–24 Years

Interventions Considered and Recommended for the Periodic Health Examination	Leading Causes of Death Motor vehicle/other unintentional injuries Homicide Suicide Malignant neoplasms Heart diseases

Interventions for the General Population

Screening
Height & Weight
Blood Pressure
Papanicolaou (Pap) test (females)
Chlamydia screen[3] (females < 20 yr.)
Rubella serology or vaccination hx[4]
  (females > 12 yr.)
Assess for problem drinking

Counseling
Injury Prevention
Lap/Shoulder Belts
Bicycle/Motorcycle/ATV helmets*
Smoke detector*
Safe storage/removal of firearms*

Substance Use
Avoid tobacco use
Avoid underage drinking and illicit drug use
Avoid alcohol/drug use while driving, swimming, boating, etc.*

Sexual Behavior
STD prevention: abstinence;* avoid high-risk behavior; condoms/female barrier with spermicide*

Diet and Exercise
Limit fat & cholesterol, maintain caloric balance, emphasize grains, fruits, vegetables
Adequate calcium intake (females)
Regular physical activity*

Dental Health
Regular visits to dental care provider*
Floss, brush with fluoride toothpaste daily

Immunization
Tetanus-diphtheria (Td) boosters (11–16 yr.)
Hepatitis B[5]
MMR (11–12 yr.)[6]
Varicella (11–12 yr.)[7]
Rubella[4] (females > 12 yr.)

CHEMOPROPHYLAXIS
Multivitamin with folic acid (females planning/capable of pregnancy)

Source: United States Preventive Services Task Force

[2]If sexually active at present or in the past: q ≤ 3 yr.   If sexual history is unreliable, begin Pap tests at age 18 yr.
[3]If sexually active.
[4]Serologic testing, documented vaccination history and routine vaccination against rubella (preferably with MMR) are equally acceptable alternatives.
[5]If not previously immunized: current visit, 1 month and 6 months later.
[6]If no previous second dose of MMR.
[7]If susceptible to chickenpox.
*The ability of clinician counseling to influence this behavior is unproven.

Table 7.2 Screening Recommendations for People Ages 25–64 Years

Interventions Considered and
Recommended for the Periodic
Health Examination

Leading Causes of Death
  Malignant neoplasms
  Heart diseases
  Motor vehicle and other unintentional
    injuries
  Human immunodeficiency virus
    (HIV) infection
  Suicide and homicide

Interventions for the General Population

Screening
Blood Pressure
Height & Weight
Total blood cholesterol (men ages 35–65,
women ages 45–85)
Papanicolaou (Pap) test (women)
Fecal occult blood test[2] and/or
  sigmoidoscopy (> 50 yr.)
Mammogram + clinical breast exam[3]
  (women 50–69 yr.)
Assess for problem drinking
Rubella serology or vaccination hx[4]
  (women of childbearing age)

Counseling

Substance Use
Tobacco cessation
Avoid alcohol/drug use while driving,
  swimming, boating, etc.

Diet and Exercise
Limit fat & cholesterol; maintain caloric
  balance; emphasize grains, fruits,
  vegetables
Adequate calcium intake (women)
Regular physical activity

Injury Prevention
Lap/shoulder belts
Motorcycle/bicycle/ATV helmets
Smoke detector
Safe storage/removal of firearms

Sexual Behavior
STD prevention: avoid high-risk behavior; condoms/female barrier with
  spermicide
Unintended pregnancy: contraception

Dental Health
Regular visits to dental care provider*
Floss, brush with fluoride toothpaste daily

Immunization
Tetanus-diphtheria (Td) boosters
Rubella[4] (women of childbearing age)

CHEMOPROPHYLAXIS
Multivitamin with folic acid (females
  planning/capable of pregnancy)
Discuss hormone prophylaxis (peri- and
  postmenopausal women)

Source: United States Preventive Services Task Force, Table 3

[1]Women who are or have been sexually active and who have a cervix: q ≤ 3 yr.
[2]Annually.
[3]Mammogram q 1–2 yr or Mammogram q 1–2 yr with annual clinical breast examination.
[4]Serologic testing, documented vaccination history and routine vaccination (preferably with
MMR) are equally acceptable alternatives.
*The ability of clinician counseling to influence this behavior is unproven.

Table 7.3　Screening Recommendations for People Age 65 and Older

Interventions Considered and Recommended for the Periodic Health Examination	Leading Causes of Death
	Heart diseases
	Malignant neoplasms (lung, colorectal, breast)
	Cerebrovascular disease
	Chronic obstructive pulmonary disease
	Pneumonia and influenza

Interventions for the General Population

Screening
Blood Pressure
Height & Weight
Fecal occult blood test[1] and/or
　sigmoidoscopy
Mammogram + clinical breast exam[2]
　(women 50–69 yr.)
Papanicolaou (Pap) test (women)[3]
Vision Screening
Assess for hearing impairment
Assess for problem drinking

Counseling

Substance Use
Tobacco cessation
Avoid alcohol/drug use while driving,
　swimming, boating, etc.

Diet and Exercise
Limit fat & cholesterol; maintain caloric
　balance; emphasize grains, fruits,
　vegetables
Adequate calcium intake (women)
Regular physical activity

Injury Prevention
Lap/shoulder belts
Motorcycle/bicycle helmets
Fall prevention
Safe storage/removal of firearms
Smoke detector
Set hot water heater to < 120–130°F
CPR training for household members

Dental Health
Regular visits to dental care provider*
Floss, brush with fluoride toothpaste daily

Sexual Behavior
STD prevention: avoid high-risk sexual
　behavior; Use condoms

Immunization
Pneumococcal vaccine
Influenza
Tetanus-diphtheria (Td) boosters

CHEMOPROPHYLAXIS
Discuss hormone prophylaxis (women)

Source: United States Preventive Services Task Force, Table 4

[1]Annually.
[2]Mammogram q 1–2 yr or Mammogram q 1–2 yr with annual clinical breast examination.
[3]All women who are or have been sexually active and who have a cervix: q ≤ 3 yr.
[4]Consider discontinuation of testing after age 65 if previous regular screening with consistently normal results.
*The ability of clinician counseling to influence this behavior is unproven.

Table 7.4   Screening Recommendations for Pregnant Women

Interventions Considered and Recommended for the
Periodic Health Examination

Interventions for the General Population

Screening
First Visit
Blood Pressure
Hemoglobin/hematocrit
Hepatitis B surface antigen (HbsAg)
RPR/VDRL
Chlamydia screen (< 25 yr.)
Rubella serology or vaccination history
D(Rh) typing, antibody screen
Offer CVS (< 13 wk)[1] or amniocentesis
  (15–18 wk)[1] (age ≥ 35 yr.)
Offer hemoglobinopathy screening
Assess for problem or risk drinking
Offer HIV screening[2]

Follow-up visits
Blood pressure
Urine culture (12–16 wk)
Offer amniocentesis (15-18 wk)[1]
  (age ≥ 35 yr.)
Offer multiple marker testing[1]
  (15–18 wk)
Offer serum α-fetoprotein[1] (16–18 wk)

Counseling
Tobacco cessation; effects of passive
  smoking
Alcohol/other drug use
Nutrition, including adequate calcium
  intake
Encourage breastfeeding
Lap/shoulder belts
Infant safety car seats
STD prevention: avoid high-risk sexual
  behavior; Use condoms

CHEMOPROPHYLAXIS
Multivitamin with folic acid[2]

Source: United States Preventive Services Task Force, Table 5
[1]Women with access to counseling and follow-up services, reliable standardized laboratories, skilled high-resolution ultrasound, and for those receiving serologic marker testing.
[2]Beginning at least 1 month before conception and continuing through the first trimester.

Secondary prevention involves screening and finding people who are at risk for chronic diseases, and early intervention while they are asymptomatic. There is tertiary prevention in the management of the disease and prevention of its complications. Adherence to therapeutic regimens, whether behavior modification, pharmacologic therapy, or both, is a cornerstone of both of these levels.

Many factors affect adherence, including the behaviors that are recommended, the complexity of the regimen, and the ease with which a patient can incorporate those recommendations into his or her daily routine. Factors that appear to significantly influence adherence include the patient's knowledge of the disease and the intervention, previous levels of adherence, confidence in his or her ability to follow recommended behaviors, perception of health and benefits of therapy or behavior, availability of social support, and complexity of the regimen. Patient empowerment and education of patient and family are key.

The American Heart Association's (AHA) expert panel on adherence found that the most promising strategies were combinations of interventions, including patient education, patient-provider learning contracts, self-monitoring, social support, and telephone follow-up.

It is important to consider two aspects of adherence: errors of omission, such as delayed and omitted doses of drug regimens, and errors of commission, such as failure to adhere to dietary and other lifestyle modifications. With few exceptions, unless the patient tells the physician or nurse about a change in lifestyle behavior or problems with carrying out recommendations, these topics are not addressed in clinical practice (Houston-Miller, 1997).

Managed care programs offer a number of advantages in chronic disease management, among them the opportunity to provide coordinated, multidisciplinary care, an appropriate frequency of office visits, short waiting times and supportive patient counseling. Despite the potential increase in costs resulting from an increase in the number of primary care visits for the management of diseases at the secondary prevention level, the total costs are lower than the aggregate of direct and indirect costs that may be avoided by reducing hospital admissions, surgical procedures and high-cost technologies (e.g., renal dialysis) (National Heart, Lung and Blood Institute, 1997).

Patients should be counseled that:

1. They are susceptible to the consequences of not following the prescribed regimen of self-care.
2. Those consequences might be severe.
3. There is a strong belief and a body of knowledge which substantiates that the benefits of the recommended self-care methods outweigh the costs and inconvenience.

Disease Management

It is important that patients play a major role in the maintenance of their own health and the management of their diseases. Disease management is an approach to patient care that coordinates medical resources for patients across the entire health care delivery system (The Boston Consulting Group, 1995). Continuous quality improvement is a core philosophy of disease management, which has four essential components: an integrated health care delivery system that is capable of coordinating health care across the continuum; a comprehensive knowledge base of the prevention, diagnosis, treatment, and palliation of disease; sophisticated clinical and administrative information systems that can be used to analyze practice patterns; and continuous quality improvement methods.

Diseases or conditions that are amenable to disease management include arthritis, asthma, chronic obstructive pulmonary disease (COPD), congestive heart failure, depression, diabetes, hypertension, hypercholesterolemia, HIV/AIDS, low back pain, and migraine headache (Coons, 1996). The criteria for the selection of diseases for disease management include:

1. High expenditures secondary to high-cost, preventable, acute events;
2. Outcomes and outcome targets that can be defined and measured in standardized and objective ways;
3. There is potential for cost savings to accrue within a short period of time; and
4. There usually is a wide variety of approaches to treating the condition, with an equally wide range of costs and outcomes (Coons, 1996).

In hypertension, for example, outcomes can be divided into three categories: immediate, which can be measured by blood pressure levels and adherence to prescribed therapeutic regimens; intermediate, which can be measured by cardiac or renal function and health resource utilization; and long-term, as measured by morbidity and mortality and the cost-effectiveness of treatment (Joint National Committee on Prevention, Detection, Evaluation, and Treatment of High Blood Pressure, 1997).

Diabetes is another example. Nationwide, although persons with diabetes represented only 4.5% of the population, the costs of diabetes therapy and the treatment of diabetic complications account for $1 out of every

$7 spent on health care (Rubin, Altman, & Mendelsohn, 1992). Non-insulin dependent diabetes mellitus (NIDDM) is the second most common principal diagnosis for office visits to internists (Barondess, 1993). Because the direct and indirect costs to the individual and to society are so great, diabetes is an ideal condition for disease management. Management of patients with diabetes mellitus or those at risk for developing it is comprised of primary prevention and diagnostic, therapeutic, and rehabilitative strategies for managing the macrovascular and microvascular sequelae (Clark & Lee, 1995).

There is primary prevention in promoting appropriate diets, physical activity, and evaluating risk factors in people who may not yet have diabetes. There is secondary prevention in terms of screening and finding people who have diabetes but are asymptomatic; and there is tertiary prevention in the management of symptomatic diabetes to prevent its complications. Patient empowerment and education of patient and family are key to its effective management. Nonetheless, only 35% of diabetic adults have attended diabetes patient education classes (Harris, 1996).

The challenge for managed care organizations is to identify those patients with diabetes who are going to cost the most and make them targets of intensive patient education efforts (Davidson, 1997). Health Maintenance Organizations (HMOs) provide a potentially beneficial environment for treating patients with chronic diseases because care can be centralized and treatment guidelines standardized, and education aimed at improving adherence can be emphasized.

The development of tailored computer-assisted instruction, expert systems, and interactive video education training adjuncts based on factors such as patients' self-identified barriers to self-management, stage of change, baseline behaviors, and social environment present new opportunities to facilitate behavior change and maintenance efficiently. Follow-up contact, either in the form of take-home materials, brief follow-up calls, support groups, and/or regular follow-up visits probably will be critical to maintaining success (Glasgow, 1995).

Medication Teaching

Prevention of iatrogenic disease is another major area where teaching is extremely important. Data from the National Health Care Survey indicate that prescriptions for medication were dispensed in six out of 10 ambulatory and seven out of 10 emergency department visits. Slightly less than half of all visits resulted in the patient receiving a prescription. The average number of prescriptions was 1.4 per person (Schappert, 1997). Among people aged 45 and over, 42% do not follow their doctor's orders when it comes to prescription medications—29% stop taking it before it is used up, and an additional 13% have their prescriptions filled but don't take the medication (American Association of Retired Persons, 1992). Although the elderly comprise 12% of the population, they account for 34% of total expenditures for prescription medications (Mueller, Schur, & O'Connell, 1997). About 11% of hospital admissions in an elderly population were found to be related to medication nonadherence, and an additional 17% resulted from adverse drug reactions (Col, Fanale, & Hornhom, 1990). An estimated $100 billion, twice the amount spent on prescription drugs, is spent annually on problems caused by nonadherence to medication regimens (Grahl, 1994). Much of the research published between 1969 and 1994 indicates that pharmacist-patient communication can improve some patient outcomes such as drug knowledge and compliance (De Young, 1996). Informing patients of potential side effects prior to starting a new medication does not lead to an increased incidence of those side effects. In fact, there is evidence that an informed patient is more likely to recognize a side effect when it occurs and thus communicate more effectively with the physician. Concern that a patient may inappropriately discontinue a medication when a side effect is suspected can be addressed by specific verbal or written instructions to the patient about what to do if a problem arises (Lamb, Green, & Heron, 1994).

With few exceptions, educating patients on how to use their medications wisely has been a missing link in our health care system. The self-administration of medication program at New York University Medical Center's Cooperative Care Center is a comprehensive education program for patients and families which involves teaching by both nurses and pharmacists (Phelan et al., 1996). Content covered in that program includes the name of each medication the patient is taking; the purpose for which it has been prescribed; the dose to be taken; frequency of administration; any significant potential side effects; when to notify a health care professional; and any special precautions to be exercised when taking the medications, including foods or drugs that should be avoided because of potential interactions. Although this program was developed for an inpatient service, its content and process can be readily adapted for ambulatory use.

Pfizer, Inc., National Healthcare Operations has developed a two part pharmacist-patient consultation program (PPCP) which is designed to train pharmacists to counsel patients about their medications and their appropriate use. This case-oriented program deals with both the physical environment of the pharmacy and the counseling area, as well as what to teach and how to teach it to patients. It stresses the need to start where the learner is, acknowledging sensory deficits, cultural and language barriers, and level of comprehension, and to recognize other patient barriers. These include: emotional displays of anger and nervousness, fear, hesitancy indicated by averted gaze, stooped posture, clenched fists, ignorance of medical terminology, senility, and developmental disability.

Pharmacists are taught that when counseling patients they should make eye contact with the patient, use an appropriate tone of voice and body language, and show the medication when talking about it. Questions to the patient should be open-ended and include active words such as who, what, how, why, when, and where. Words such as can, do, did, does, will, have, are, and would should not be used.

The Omnibus Budget Reconciliation Act of 1990 (OBRA '90) mandated that pharmacists counsel patients on the following points:

1. The name and description of the medication;
2. The dosage form, dose, route of administration, and duration of drug therapy;
3. Special directions and precautions for preparation, administration, and use by the patient;
4. Common (severe) side effects or adverse effects or interactions and therapeutic contraindications that may be encountered, including their avoidance and the action required if they occur;
5. Techniques for self-monitoring drug therapy;
6. Proper storage;
7. Prescription refill information; and
8. Actions to be taken in the event of a missed dose.

On December 1, 1998 the Food and Drug Administration established a requirement that certain products that pose a serious and significant threat to public health bear Agency-approved labels that contain necessary information for patients to use their medications safely and effectively. The regulation became effective June 1, 1999. Required information includes why the product poses a serious and significant public health concern, the product's indications for use, contraindications, directions for use, precautions, and possible side effects. There also must be a statement that a drug product should not be used for a condition other than the one for which it was prescribed.

Teaching Methods

Verbal counseling should be supplemented by specific written information about each drug, a procedure followed by most pharmacies. MedTeach for Windows, a product of the American Society of Health-System Pharmacists, is one program which can generate this type of information. In cases where patients have limited reading ability or use a language other than English, a chart can be made with each pill pasted on it, along with the name (if only for others to identify), a simple one- or two-word explanation of what the medication is for (e.g., water for a diuretic or a picture of a heart for cardiotonic medications), a clock indicating the hours when it should be taken and a picture of food (if it should be taken with food). While this is less than ideal, it is far better than nothing. Audiotapes and, where available, videotapes also can be used to achieve this purpose.

To enhance this factual information, we recommend that open-ended questions be asked of patients such as:

1. What did the doctor tell you the medication is for?
2. How did the doctor tell you to take the medication?
3. What did the doctor tell you to expect?

Patients should be asked to repeat the answers for a final verification.

Counseling for Lifestyle Change

The United States Preventive Services Task Force recommends the following strategies for counseling patients:

1. *Frame the teaching to match the patient's perceptions.* To enhance self-efficacy identify the patient' beliefs that are relevant to the behavior, start where the patient is, and provide information based upon this foundation.

2.   *Fully inform patients of the purposes and expected effects of interventions and when to expect these effects.* Patients need to know how long it will take for the effects of interventions to become evident. For example, they need to be told that the maximum effect of exercise on lowering cholesterol can take as much as a year or two. If prescribed medications cause side effects they should be told what to expect, and under what circumstances the provider should be consulted or they should stop taking the medication.

3.   *Suggest small changes rather than large ones.* Patients with elevated cholesterol who consume diets that are high in animal fat should be encouraged to try having meatless Mondays rather than admonished to become near vegetarians overnight. Exercise also may be introduced in the form of taking a fifteen minute walk, perhaps as a family, after dinner on most nights when the weather is decent. The amount of exercise can be increased gradually over time as the patient begins to see and reap its benefits and enjoy the process.

4.   *Be specific.* "Get some exercise" or "Cut way back on your fat" without having a sense of the patient's baseline and establishing some specific interim goals is not likely to meet with success.

5.   *It is sometimes easier to add new behaviors than to eliminate established ones.* Obese patients may respond better to the introduction of an exercise regimen than the imposition of a strict diet.

6.   *Link new behaviors to old established ones.* Taking a walk after dinner, or taking one's daily aspirin with breakfast may help the new habit to become internalized sooner.

7.   *Use the power of the profession.* Patients, especially older ones, view health professionals, especially physicians as experts. Even those who have more collegial relationships are likely to see the provider as a consultant. Some if not all patients will respond positively to simple directives to reduce the fat in their diets by one-half or to quit smoking. In issuing such edicts, however, the clinician should be empathetic and supportive and acknowledge that some patients may lack confidence in their ability to make lifestyle changes.

8.   *Get explicit commitments from the patient.* Sedentary adults who need to get exercise can promise to take 15–20 minute walks with their families after dinner at least three times a week. On days when they don't do this get them to commit to getting off the bus a stop further from work than they normally do or park at the far end of the lot. Instead of imposing rigid diets to lower cholesterol, get the patient to commit to giving up red meat or butter and replace it with vegetables. At the next visit ask the patient to modify a bit more.

9. *Use a combination of strategies.* Individual counseling should be supplemented by group educational sessions or support groups, appropriate use of audiovisual aids and written materials.

10. *Involve office staff.* Everyone in the office has a patient education responsibility. Even the receptionist has a role in encouraging patients to read the materials in the reception area. If the practice is large you can offer educational programs, send out a newsletter, and establish a patient resource library. Having a patient education committee is a good idea.

11. *Refer.* Patients can be referred to community agencies, national voluntary health organizations, such as the American Diabetes Association, instructional references such as books, audio and video tapes, and, where appropriate, websites, and role models. Patients who have the same problem, have made changes, and are doing well can be potent motivators for individuals who need to change their behaviors.

12. *Monitor progress through follow-up contact.* Schedule a follow-up appointment or telephone call within a relatively short interval to evaluate progress, reinforce success, and identify and respond to problems. This can substantially improve the effectiveness of clinical counseling (USPSTF, lxvii–lxxx).

In addressing how providers can adapt their practices for health promotion, Westberg and Jason suggest the following steps:

1. Formulate goals for your practice.
2. Decide on your approach to patients.
3. Decide how you and your colleagues can function as a team.
4. Have visible signs of the emphasis on health promotion.
5. Select and use systems and resources that support your team's health promotion efforts.
6. Select and use systems and resources that support your patients' health promotion efforts.
7. Have a member of the team coordinate special health promotion efforts.

Suggestions for addressing health behavior issues with patients include:

1. Be sure that patients understand the reasons for addressing health behavior.
2. Discuss how you can work as partners in addressing their health issues.
3. Help them explore their health-related behaviors and identify their risk factors.

4. Explore their attitudes about key risk factors.

5. Help them explore factors that have the potential to support and obstruct their efforts to change.

6. Try to facilitate their commitments to making positive changes.

7. Help them establish realistic goals.

8. Help them develop workable plans for achieving their goals.

9. Work with patients in monitoring their progress.

10. Schedule follow-up visits and telephone calls with patients after they achieve their goals, especially those that are difficult to sustain.

11. Be patient with your own and your patients' efforts to make significant changes.

In teaching patients the knowledge, skills, and attitudes needed for primary, secondary, or tertiary prevention, it is important to assess their level of involvement in the desired behavioral change. It also is important to help them accept "lapses" and "relapses" in their behavior as part of the process of moving to healthier behaviors. Prochaska has provided us with a model of self-directed behavioral change that is extremely useful for understanding and communicating this process. In it people move through a series of stages as follows: precontemplation, contemplation, action, maintenance, and relapse. They can move back and forth through the stages. By assessing where your patient is in this cycle, you can focus your education on the proper issues. You also can avoid wasting time giving someone who does not believe that change is important a plan for change, and focus instead on developing his or her motivation and seeking to reduce the harm which is likely to result from the failure to control unhealthy habits.

Chapter 8
The Frail Elderly

Eugenia L. Siegler and Adeboye Francis

Clinicians in private practice may be reluctant to care for frail elderly because these patients have complex medical, social, emotional, and functional problems. Providers may feel unable to meet all of these needs under the best of circumstances; when managed care incentives impose time constraints that limit basic clinical assessment, supplemental patient and family education would seem impossible even to contemplate. Nonetheless, effective management of the frail patient necessitates clinical care and patient and family education in all of these domains. This chapter will describe methods that clinicians can use to help family and patient cope with illness and disability.

Frailty—What It Is, and Why It Causes Disability

When asked to imagine what it means to be frail, most people have a visceral response, envisioning someone at the end of life, and often imbuing the image with a sense of hopelessness. In the gerontologic literature, physical frailty is defined as "severely impaired strength, mobility, balance, and endurance" (Hadley, Ory, Suzman, & Weindruch, 1989). This medical definition seems to lack the emotional content that underlies a lay definition, but the two meanings share the same implications of dependency and functional decline. The medical definition of frailty, however, offers hope of intervention and reversibility, and clinical trials have been designed to reduce physical dependence by concentrating on the components of frailty (Ory, Schechtman, Miller, & Hadley, 1993). The clinician should keep the medical definition in mind when working with the frail elderly patient and family. The situation is not hopeless, and there is much that the clinician can do to improve the patient's medical and functional status. Education, in particular, can serve both preventive and rehabilitative purposes.

Demographics of Enrollment in Managed Care Programs That Serve the Elderly

Although most elderly are not significantly impaired, clinicians can anticipate that the majority of their frail patients will be elderly Medicare recipients. Medicare enrollment is increasing, reflecting the growth in the nation's elderly population. Since 1975, the number of Medicare recipients over 65 has increased by almost 50%, to 33.6 million (Table 8.1).

The population of Medicare enrollees is heterogeneous, spanning many decades and reflecting the nation's ethnic diversity (Table 8.2). This heterogeneity will have an impact on the range of health status that the clinician might see in a Medicare population, as well as the patient and family responses to illness and impairment.

The growth of managed care Medicare and Medicaid plans is a more recent phenomenon, but managed care plans already account for more than 10% of Medicare enrollees. As of May, 1997, 4.6 million elderly

Table 8.1   Medicare and Medicaid Recipients/Trends for People 65 and Over

	Fiscal Year					
	1975	1980	1985	1995	1996	1997
	In millions					
Medicare	22.8	25.5	28.2	33.0	33.4	33.6
Medicaid	3.6	3.4	3.1	4.2	4.4	4.6

Years 1995–1997 are estimated for Medicaid data; Years 1996 and 1997 are estimated for Medicare data

Source: www.HCFA.gov/stats/hstats9/blustats.htm#trend

Table 8.2 Medicare Enrollment/Demographics

	Total	Male	Female
	In thousands		
All persons	37,829	16,205	21,623
Aged	33,264	13,502	19,762
65–74	18,104	8,079	10,025
75–84	11,255	4,342	6,913
85 years +	3,905	1,081	2,824
White	32,368	13,819	18,549
Black	3,382	1,438	1,944
All other	1,662	786	877
Native American	35	18	17
Asian/Pacific	180	78	101
Hispanic	427	209	217
Other	1,021	480	541
Unknown race	417	163	254

Source: www.HCFA.gov/stats/hstats9/blustats.htm#trend

Table 8.3 Medicare Managed Care Programs

	Number of Plans	Enrollees in thousands
Total prepaid	274	3,814
Health Care Prepayment plans or Group Practice prepayment plans	56	523
TEFRA risk	181	3,089
Cost Basis	32	183
Demonstrations	5	19
Percentage of total Medicare Beneficiaries		10.0

Source: www.HCFA.gov/stats/hstats9/blustats.htm#trend

were enrolled in Medicare risk contract HMOs (Management, 1998). Earlier chapters have described the nature and types of managed care plans. Table 8.3 demonstrates that Medicare-based programs have taken a variety of forms.

The Health Care Financing Administration (HCFA) has funded many demonstration projects, in addition to the more typical Medicare risk-based plans. These have tested less traditional systems of caring for the elderly, such as Social Health Maintenance Organizations (S/HMOs) or Programs of All Inclusive Care for the Elderly (PACE). Thus, although there are justifiable concerns about the effects of managed care on the physician-patient relationship, especially as capitation and lower fees have increased pressures to limit encounter time, some of the most innovative care systems for the elderly have been "managed." For many elderly, managed care has brought significant improvement in quality of life, and overzealous criticisms of managed care often fail to acknowledge this.

This chapter will briefly describe some innovative programs only as examples of what is possible; unfortunately, relatively few elderly and physicians can participate in these plans. Most of the chapter will describe methods that providers can use to simultaneously educate frail elderly and their families and maintain efficient practices while participating in the more common Medicare managed care plans.

Innovative Managed Care Programs

Social Health Maintenance Organizations (S/HMOs) and Program of All Inclusive Care for the Elderly (PACE) models are capitated programs funded by special waivers from HCFA and/or state Medicaid programs to meet the acute and long-term care (LTC) needs of frailest elders; these programs all incorporate social and educational elements. PACE programs, for example (Branch, Coulam, & Zimmerman, 1995; Eng, Pedulla, Eleazer, McCann, & Fox, 1997) focus on patients dually eligible for Medicare and Medicaid, and must have an adult day care component; this setting is ideal for patient education. These programs are growing in number and scope, and they target the frailest elderly, those who would otherwise qualify for nursing home care; unfortunately, the number of patients who can enroll in them is limited—usually several hundred per site.

S/HMOs originally targeted a broader case mix, and were "equivalent to a Medicare risk-based HMO to which a modest private LTC insurance policy had been grafted" (Kane et al., 1997, p. 102). In their first trials in the 1980s, S/HMOs failed to demonstrate any added advantage to existing Medicare HMOs. Now in their second "generation," S/HMOs are being redesigned to practice evidence-based geriatric care and improve LTC benefits (Kane et al., 1997).

Most physicians do not work in these special kinds of managed care systems and thus have no access to the social and educational innovations that these programs have offered. Instead, providers must supply their own teaching or encourage HMOs to create these kinds of programs.

The First Educational Step: Helping Patients Choose a Capitated Plan

The first responsibility of the provider is to educate the patient and family about managed care itself—whether to choose a plan, how the plans work, etc. Usually, the elderly do have a choice—if they are not working or dependent on retirement benefits, they can opt either for "straight" Medicare or for one of the Medicare managed care plans. For those without Medicaid or Medigap insurance, Medicare managed care plans are very appealing, and wholesale condemnation will serve little purpose. Staff can be trained to discuss the options with patients, and the provider is well advised to spend a few minutes answering patients' questions about the benefits and disadvantages of managed care plans. Counseling patients and family who are worried about escalating costs of chronic illness will enhance the provider-patient relationship through times of financial stress.

Clinicians can begin by offering guidelines for choosing managed care plans that are elderly-friendly. HCFA has an Internet site about managed care (Table 8.4) to which the clinician can refer the patient or from which

Table 8.4   Selected Internet Web Sites Relevant to Elderly and Their Caregivers

AHCPR Guidelines	www.ahcpr.gov/consumer/
Administration on Aging	www.aoa.dhhs.gov/elderpage.htm
Caregiving	www.caregiving.com/support/html/links.htm
Medicare	www.medicare.gov/index.asp
Managed Care	www.medicare.gov/managedcare.html#compar
General education	www.healthfinder.gov
	www.uic.edu/depts/lib/health/hw/consumer/internet.html
	www.aoa.dhhs.gov:80/aoa/webres/swsab.htm

the office staff can download materials to maintain as hard copy. In addition, the HMO Workgroup on Care Management recently published a set of guidelines specifying what services should be available to older individuals enrolled in Medicare managed care plans (Management, 1998). Although some of these recommendations relate to quality and data management, others are more relevant to patient care and education and include:

Systematic programs to identify high risk enrollees

- Mechanisms to identify and coordinate social services
- Geriatric case management services in all settings
- Geriatric expertise for administration and consultation
- Geriatric education and training for staff and physicians
- Wellness programs
- Educational programs for elderly and caregivers

To assist patients who wish to leave fee-for-service Medicare and join a Medicare HMO, providers may share the guidelines as an aid to making an informed choice. However, at the time of this writing, Medicare HMOs are pulling back on their services, and interest among seniors appears to be on the decline.

Educating About Health and Illness

When talking with patients and family, the clinician must consider two extra factors: The role of the caregiver, and the multiplicity of illnesses.

The Caregiver

Although patients of any age and ability may request that the clinician provide information to trusted family members and may wish that family members be involved in decision making, family members may be obliged to assume the larger and more crucial role of caregiver in the lives of the frail elderly.

Clinicians must determine who should receive the education—caregiver, patient, or both. When an elderly patient and relative are both in the examination or consultation room, clinicians must resist the temptation to address the caregiver first. Effective communication with the elderly and their families begins with respect, and even if the patient is demented or the caregiver is the primary source of information, the clinician will best demonstrate respect by addressing and questioning the patient first. After a brief exchange, the clinician can then determine if the patient is too demented or too physically dependent to absorb information.

In addition, caregivers have their own needs. Effective education necessitates some understanding of the caregiver's role and how caregiving responsibilities are managed logistically, emotionally, and financially.

The Multiplicity of Medical Problems

The provider may feel overwhelmed trying to teach patient and caregiver when the frail elderly patient may have five or six medical problems, 10 medications, and dependencies in several activities of daily living. Yet these patients and caregivers require the most education and support. The clinician must determine patient and caregiver priorities and incorporate educational strategies as part of the evaluation.

Patient and Caregiver Education: One Approach

Case Study

An 80-year-old African-American man was brought to the office by his daughter, who said he was falling at least twice a month. He denied loss of consciousness, palpitations, head trauma, and lightheadedness. No seizure activity had been noted. He had had multiple visits to the Emergency room for suturing of lacerations and soft tissue trauma.

The patient lived with his daughter, because he was unable to care for himself alone after the death of his wife. His past medical history was notable for hypertension, severe degenerative joint disease, coronary artery disease, status post coronary artery bypass grafting, and mild-moderate dementia of at least 3 years' duration. His medications were: aspirin; metoprolol 50 mg twice daily; diphenhydramine 50 mg at bedtime; and acetaminophen 650 mg, every 6 hours as needed. He did not smoke or drink.

On physical examination, he was a pleasant, healthy-appearing elderly man, in no obvious distress. Vital signs were all within normal limits. He was not orthostatic. Pertinent physical findings included a resolving hematoma over the left buttock, an S4 gallop, and an enlarged prostate. His gait was wide-based with a shortened stride, and he was most unsteady during turns and when rising from a chair. There were no localizing signs on neurological examination. Tone was mildly increased throughout, and he had some loss of sensation in both lower extremities. His Mini Mental Status exam score was 19/30.

Comment

Situations like this can be overwhelming for patient, caregiver, and clinician alike. The clinician must assess the status of the patient's underlying medical conditions; determine the cause of the falls, which requires assessment of patient-related, treatment-related, and environmental factors; evaluate and adjust medications; determine the safety of the home environment and access social services, if necessary; ascertain the patient's level of comprehension and tailor counseling to meet the patient's needs; and educate the caregiver about all of these problems, while at the same time offering reassurance and encouragement.

How does the PCP allocate the 30–45 minutes allowed for a new patient encounter? It is best to begin by establishing mutual goals. Here, the caveat about caregiver concerns is in force. When taking the history, the clinician must quickly learn what the patient's and caregiver's goals are, how they differ, and how to reconcile them. The PCP must then establish a problem list that incorporates these goals and respects patient and caregiver priorities.

The clinician who is fortunate enough to practice with nurses, social workers, and other nonphysician providers can share many of the assessment and educational responsibilities with them. For those who practice alone, fitting education and counseling into the clinical encounter requires a talent for multitasking.

Begin with the Functional Assessment

Caregivers and patients are concerned about how they will cope with their impairments, and understanding how the patient functions is essential to teaching what the patient and caregiver need to know. The functional domains are divided into the Activities of Daily Living (ADL) and the Instrumental Activities of Daily Living (IADL). ADL include essential tasks such as bathing, dressing, feeding, toileting, and mobility skills such as ambulation and transferring. IADL are more sophisticated tasks, such as housekeeping, managing finances or medications, and using the telephone or transportation. Many articles describe basic approaches to functional assessment (Applegate, Blass, & Williams, 1990; Lachs et al., 1990).

Functional assessment serves many purposes: it helps determine what the patient's needs are; it provides assessment of the impact of disease on the patient's life; and, most importantly for the purposes of patient education, it allows the patient (and/or caregiver) to articulate priorities. What is most important to the patient—independence in ambulation, minimization of medications, living independently, or energy conservation? How much can the patient comprehend, and what role does the patient want to play in decision making? The functional assessment allows the clinician to assess the degree of frailty and engage patient and caregiver in the treatment process at the same time.

For this patient, functional assessment will determine where the patient needs help and what he wishes to do on his own, and it may provide insight into the cause of the falls. For example, is he insistent on being as independent as possible, and are the falls related to his unsuccessful attempts to perform IADL activities like housekeeping tasks? Are there conflicts over what the patient and his daughter feel that he can do safely? Does he experience episodes of dizziness when transferring or attempting to get to the bathroom?

Acknowledge the Caregiver's Needs and Contributions

Caregivers have real needs and fears. They want to do a good job, and they often fear that they are not adequately serving their loved one. Most have no experience in a health profession, and they may not even know what questions to ask, or may be too embarrassed to ask them.

In a study of educational needs of caregivers of adults who had recently become disabled, Weeks (1995) found that the highest priority was to learn to "normalize the daily routine of a disabled adult within the bounds of his or her disabilities" (p. 259). Other areas that caregivers felt especially important to learn were ensuring that assistance was available, evaluating functional capacity, ensuring that treatment plans were followed, and anticipating the loved one's future needs (Mathis, 1989). Acknowledgment of these needs and reassurance of the caregiver at the time of the patient evaluation will engage the caregiver and increase the likelihood that the caregiver will communicate needs and follow through on the clinician's advice.

This patient's daughter has taken him into her home because of worsening cognitive and functional status. She has lost privacy and leisure time, and she has added anxiety over her father's health. She will require honest explanations of the medical issues, especially the cognitive impairment and the contribution that his medications may be making to cognitive and gait impairment. She will also want enough information to be able to anticipate future problems, and she will benefit from support, praise, and encouragement in her role as caregiver. Some of this can occur during the history or in the final summary after physical examination, but clinicians need not devote too much time to details during the first encounter; the patients and caregivers can absorb only limited amounts of information at a time, and the clinician should make it clear that the relationship with patient and family is an ongoing one which is not just limited to the diagnostic process. Advice, information, and support should be parceled out over time, because although frail patients' and caregivers' needs change, there are always needs that the clinician must meet.

Teach While Observing the Patient

The examination of the frail elderly patient often involves observation of gait, inspection or care of skin, and evaluation of neurologic deficits. Unlike cardiac auscultation, these evaluations can be interactive and are perfect opportunities for instruction. For example, involving the caregiver in skin evaluation to demonstrate at-risk areas, such as sacrum or occiput, and proper wound care techniques combines patient evaluation/management and education.

In the case of this patient, the history of multiple falls necessitates a thorough evaluation of gait and balance. The clinician can watch the patient as he comes into the office, sits down in the chair, rises to go to the examination table, or descends from the table. Tandem gait, toe and heel walking, and turning can be substituted for manual muscle testing, and they allow the clinician both to assess the patient and to educate the patient and caregiver about hazardous maneuvers and situations most likely to lead to a fall.

Providers also can instruct patients like this one in the proper use of a cane or walker as they watch patients walk; they can ask about tripping hazards at home or inquire about episodes of instability; and they can make suggestions about minimizing fall hazards during the examination.

Provide Explanations During the History

Caregivers of demented patients will report problem behaviors. When taking the history, the provider can explain the behavior and its meaning, and as part of the process can offer coping mechanisms. It is best to take a history from the caregiver separately from the patient physical examination, to allow the caregiver to freely express concerns and describe problem behaviors. Finding the appropriate time can be difficult; often, speaking with the caregiver for 5–10 minutes over the phone a day or two before the visit will suffice, and will allow the provider to spend the office visit efficiently, examining and reassuring the patient.

In the case of this patient, discussing the circumstances under which the patient came to live with her will provide insight into the degree of cognitive impairment and its clinical manifestations. Explaining the nature of dementia and the reasons for the decline will help the daughter accept and understand the dementia, and will at the same time communicate to her that the PCP acknowledges the dementia and shares her concerns.

Offer References and Web Addresses

Innumerable resources are available in book and pamphlet form, and on the Internet. Patients and caregivers may need some assistance and advice when trying to find information (Ahmed & Siegler, 1997). Table 8.4 lists some of the more comprehensive World Wide Web pages that cover topics relevant to the elderly.

Clinicians who do not specialize in care of frail elderly may lack sufficient experience with dementing illnesses to feel comfortable advising patients and family members about coping with the illness. These references can save time and supplement clinician advice. Patients and families also may be reluctant to "bother" clinicians, and having references at home may both reassure them and spare clinicians follow-up phone calls for information about behavioral or other problems.

Take Advantage of "The Aging Network"

Since 1965, a number of organizations that serve the elderly or that have received federal funding through the Older Americans Act have been linked together to form a loosely organized structure called "The Aging Network" (Administration on Aging [AoA], 1998). Strictly defined, The Network includes the Administration on Aging, also known as the AoA (federal); state units on aging; Area Agencies on Aging, also known as AAAs (county); and organizations that provide services for them, such as Meals on Wheels, senior centers, case management programs, ombudsman and legal services programs, Title IV demonstration projects, and Title VI and VII tribal programs (Kane & Baker, 1996). Others take a broader view of The Network and include voluntary organizations and academic gerontologic and geriatric programs (AoA, 1998).

Exactly how the Aging Network will respond to managed care is a subject of some debate and reflects the many roles of the network—long-term care ombudsman, care management, education, nutrition, and consumer advocacy, to name a few (Kane & Baker, 1996). Although somewhat diminished due to funding cuts, the Network remains a useful resource. As loosely organized as it is, the Network is organized, and entry into any one area can provide access to other organizations. The Network's linkages have fostered their World Wide Web counterparts, and these web sites provide quick access to information about services and programs for the elderly. On The Aging Network's web page, for example, are URLs for aging resources and directories to organizations that are part of the Network. Providers can offer the URLs or download information about local agencies to share with patients and families (AoA, 1998).

Encourage Caregivers and Patients to Join Support Groups

There are support groups for virtually every disease, and many that deal with chronic illnesses, such as Alzheimer's disease focus on the caregiver. Support groups are an invaluable source of peer education, advice, and emotional sustenance. These groups are especially useful when patients or caregivers have questions about specific difficult situations and they require practical, real-world advice.

The Internet is another potential source of support. Because they may have hundreds or even thousands of subscribers, listservs, for example, can provide an even broader range of advice than can real-time support groups. They also offer the advantage of convenience. The subscriber need never leave the house and can log on at any time. For this patient's daughter, peer advice and support, whether "real time" or via a listserv, can be an outstanding source of education and advice.

Incorporate Advance Directives into the Initial Assessment

Elderly patients will welcome discussions of advance directives. A brief, early investment in having the patient designate a health care representative who knows the patient's wishes about mechanical ventilation, tube feedings and resuscitation will save many more emotionally charged and hurried conversations later. Clinicians should become familiar with their state's laws regarding living wills, durable powers of attorney, and other forms of advance directives. Most of the paperwork need not involve the clinician at all, as long as he or she documents the discussion in the chart and spends a few moments with the patient and caregiver reassuring them that their wishes are understood and will be followed. Staff can help patients prepare health care representative forms (depending on individual state laws) and can witness the signatures; providers can use these as a stepping-off point for beginning the discussion about more delicate issues.

This patient, although demented, is able to give a history and can understand what it means to choose a health care representative. Explaining to the family and patient the importance of advance planning is "now" reassures them that the clinician is interested in following their wishes, and encourages them to make decisions at a time that they can be made thoughtfully and carefully. This kind of discussion need take only a few minutes, as the patient and caregiver usually will want to spend some time at home thinking about the options. Their decisions can then be discussed at a follow-up visit and documented in the chart.

Advantages of S/HMOs and PACE Programs

The previous discussion has presupposed that the clinician practices without the assistance of non-physician providers. The physician decides if the patient needs assistance from nursing, social work, or physical therapists, and accesses them via existing channels, such as an outpatient rehabilitation unit or a Certified Home Health Agency. The more experimental managed care programs have incorporated these services as part of the care system. In a S/HMO program, for example, the patient would have a care manager who would obtain and coordinate services of nursing, social work, physical therapists, and others according to the physician's directions. The S/HMO personnel would assist with care coordination between acute and community settings. To be eligible for a PACE program, the patient would have to be "nursing home certifiable" that is, impaired enough to qualify for nursing home care. If the patient belonged to a PACE program, an interdisciplinary team would evaluate him, meet, and create his plan of care. Thus, the team would determine the educational needs and the means to meet them, whether through home visits, in a clinician's office, or as part of an adult day care program (Eng et al., 1997). Both of these scenarios facilitate patient education by recognizing the importance of the patient's social and educational needs and by including care management (which facilitates access to nonphysician providers) as an essential component.

Conclusion

For the busy clinician, managed care pressures to limit encounter time can make caring for frail elderly an impossible task. Education of frail elderly and caregivers can be effective if it is combined with assessment and if clinicians take advantage of the systems that are already in place. That frailty has so many dimensions beyond the medical can be either an endless frustration or a tremendous relief to the busy clinician. Clinicians who try to do all of the educating, or who limit their teaching to the strictly medical, will almost certainly fail; those who acknowledge and embrace the multidimensional nature of education can assist and encourage patients and caregivers to learn both in and outside the office.

Chapter 9

Asthma

Joan Reibman, Cara Cassino, and
Wendy Berkowitz

Epidemiology

Asthma affects approximately 14 million people in the United States and is one of the most common diseases managed by the primary care physician (Mannino et al., 1998). In the 14-year period from 1980–1994, the annual age-adjusted prevalence rate of self-reported asthma increased 75%, with an increase in the death rate of 20% (Mannino et al., 1998). In 1995, there were more than 1.8 million emergency room visits for asthma as a first-listed diagnosis (Mannino et al., 1998). Asthma is the single most common cause of a hospital visit in children. In 1990, the cost of illness related to asthma was estimated at 6.2 billion dollars including direct medical expenditures of 1.6 billion dollars for in-patient services and 200 million dollars for emergency room visits (Weiss et al., 1992).

Although many possibilities have been suggested for the increase in morbidity, poor education and limited access to care have been implicated as major roles in the increase.

Difficulties in the Management of Asthma

There are numerous obstacles to optimal care of a patient with asthma. These may include environmental problems, such as elevated levels of ambient pollutants, workplace exposures, and poor living conditions with mold, rodent, and cockroach infestation. Moreover, social problems may aggravate management difficulties.

Importance of Education in Asthma Management

Specific characteristics of asthma make it a disease that necessitates intensive and repeated educational efforts (Table 9.1).

Disease Chronicity and Variability

Asthma is a chronic disease, and management aims at the prevention of symptoms. However, the variable and often unpredictable course of asthma can result in dramatic variation in the severity of the disease. This characteristic causes many management difficulties, since adherence tends to be affected by the patient's perception of the severity of the illness.

Changing Medications with Disease Activity

The chronicity and variability of asthma make vigilance a necessity and require that regimens be continuously tailored to disease activity. Often, patients are adherent with prescribed regimens during and immediately after acute exacerbations. However, when their symptoms have improved, they may find it difficult to accept that they still have a disease which requires regular use of certain medications for prevention. They may start to resume their usual activities and, because they feel well, become nonadherent to monitoring and the use of prophylactic medications. In-

---

Table 9.1   Characteristics of Asthma that Necessitate Education

- Disease chronicity
- Disease variability
- Changing medication regimens with disease activity
- Complexity of medication regimens
- High level of nonadherence to medical regimens
- Potential for self-management

creases in disease activity may be overlooked. The stage is then set for an asthma exacerbation. Thus, the variability of the disease course fosters denial of disease, and poses a particular problem to the health care provider who is educating the patient and family about asthma (Kohler et al., 1995). The chronicity and variability of the disease is a critical issue to explain to patients and, particularly, to their families. Chronicity demands that teaching be repeated regularly. Because of the variability of the disease, education must be used to reinforce continuous vigilance. Success in this endeavor requires a partnership between the patient and provider.

Complexity of Medication Regimens

A major difficulty in the management of asthma lies in the ability and desire of a patient to adhere to prescribed therapy. Indeed, studies have demonstrated that at most, 50% of patients take their medications at a therapeutic dose (Cockrane, 1998; Marinker, 1998; Rand et al., 1992).

Difficulties with Adherence to Medical Regimens

Failure of adherence to prescribed medications may be due to: (1) failure to obtain the medication; (2) intentional disregard of the recommendations; or (3) unintentional disregard. It is important to determine whether any of these reasons underly a patient's noncompliance with therapy, as interventions may be available. For example, the failure of a patient to obtain the medication may be due to practical difficulties, such as inability to afford it, inability to get to a pharmacy, or unavailability at the local pharmacy. Intentional failure to take the medication may be due to denial and rejection of the disease. Should this be the problem, socially and culturally appropriate education efforts may be focused on these issues. Unintentional noncompliance may be due to multiple clinical, social, and psychological causes. These issues need to be recognized and, when possible, additional services may be recommended to the patient (Cockrane, 1998; Marinker, 1998).

Potential for Self-Management

Working with the patient to develop realistic short- and long-term management goals during visits improves asthma management (Clark et al., 1995).

These goals can be developed to include individualized self-management programs.

When to Teach

Teachable Moments

Several techniques are helpful when teaching a patient about asthma. One of these makes use of the variability of the disease and the concept of a "teachable moment," a time when a patient is both receptive to information and available.

Recovery After an Acute Event

Often, a patient is most receptive to learning about asthma after an acute event, when the fear of another episode is greatest. Thus, the recovery period during a hospitalization for asthma affords a prototypical "teachable moment." At this time patients usually are still receiving medication, have been frightened, and are concerned about their disease. They also are available.

Office/Clinic Visit

Waiting time before being seen by the health care provider should be used for an educational intervention. The difficulty with this approach lies in the varying time available and the concern a patient may have that he or she will miss being called by the physician. However, with reassurance, this time can be used with great benefit. Clearly, the visit with the health care provider is an optimal time for an education and face-to-face encounters with the health care provider are an excellent means of teaching. However, particularly in today's medical environment, visits may be rushed and may not allow for the time that a good educational session requires. Regardless, specific issues should be reviewed or reinforced at each visit with a stepwise approach to instruction.

Following Office/Clinic Visit

A planned session after the visit with the provider, when the patient no longer is anxious about being seen and is more clear about the medical condition, also may serve as an excellent moment for instruction. Additional advantages are that the patient already is on-site and does not need to make a special trip. A visit with a nurse or educator can be scheduled for this time. The disadvantages are that the visit is prolonged, and the patient may be anxious to leave, or overloaded with information.

During an Emergency Visit

An emergent visit also may be an excellent time for teaching. However, there are few health care professionals with the time, training, or dedication to use this time in most busy emergency centers, and the setting of a bustling, noisy emergency department may be less than optimal for a calm educational intervention. In addition, the patient may be anxious and fearful, making him or her less receptive to instruction. Nevertheless, using a dedicated asthma educator and a focused intervention, we have used this time successfully to reinforce the concept of early warning signals of asthma that may predate an emergency room visit, and the need for ambulatory follow-up (Godoy et al., 1998).

Scheduled Educational Sessions

Finally, special sessions may be scheduled for the patient. This approach is excellent because it affords the patient a calm, organized, formal series of sessions. However, repeated studies have demonstrated that cooperation with this approach takes a dedicated patient, and many patients do not return for these visits. In addition, extra transportation costs and sometimes visit charges, which could serve as a deterrent, may be incurred.

Our tactic has been to use multiple techniques, and in our urban hospital we now have educational sessions designed for the emergency department, inpatient stay, and before and after a clinic visit. Because of the barriers mentioned above, we have not extensively requested that patients come for separate sessions. An overview of potential "teachable moments" is outlined in Table 9.2.

Who Should Teach

Education can be performed by a variety of personnel including physicians, nurses, respiratory therapists, and pharmacists, as well as peer health educators.

Physician

The most effective way to transmit information is during a face-to-face encounter between the patient, family, and provider. However, if the physician is pressed for time, it is important to identify specific issues that need to be addressed immediately and to focus on them. Time should be taken to elicit patients' concerns and perceptions about their asthma.

Table 9.2   Choosing a Teachable Moment

Moment	Advantages	Disadvantages
During the wait for an office/clinic visit	Receptive patient	Variable time
After an office/clinic visit	Patient already at location	Extends visit, patient anxious to leave, get prescriptions filled, etc.
During an ED visit	Receptive patient	Anxiety may preclude attention and information retention
Special scheduled education session	Receptive patient	Necessity of extra trip, extra transportation cost, may preclude attendance
During a hospitalization	Bored, receptive patient	Not all patients hospitalized, patient anxious during acute event, need trained hospital personnel
Off-site: Pharmacy, community program, school	Convenient locale, culturally familiar	Difficult to organize

Retention of material reviewed may not be great because of the anxiety a patient may have during a visit with a physician. Adjunctive educational material to reinforce the teaching points can be used in such situations.

Nurse Educator or Health Educator

A specially trained asthma nurse or health educator can provide additional educational support. The patient may not be as anxious with a nurse, and there may be more time available. Teaching can be done individually or in group sessions with an educational leader. The discussion that ensues may lead to the disclosure of additional problems, and patients can teach and learn from one another.

Respiratory Therapist

Depending on their training, respiratory therapists are increasingly being used as health educators. Their educational role is being stressed more frequently in current training programs.

Pharmacist

Pharmacists are increasingly involved as educators. Although they are the most frequent source of advice for patients, they often have been overlooked by health care providers as a source of patient educational information.

Each educator may reinforce different components, and each should be used in the sphere of his or her expertise. For example a respiratory therapist may best be used to teach the techniques of the use of devices such as large volume spacers, nebulizers or peak flow meters. However, it would be inappropriate for them to explain pharmacologic management. A pharmacist can explain the role and side effects of medications. Education by an allied health care professional should be used to reinforce a medical regimen developed by the primary health care provider. Care must be taken to train the educator to direct questions outside the sphere of his or her expertise to the appropriate person. Optimally, specific issues can be taught in one setting and reinforced in another. Exposure to different teaching approaches may enhance understanding of a topic. Regardless of the technique used, concepts need to be repeated regularly, and patients should be asked to demonstrate continued ability to perform skills at subsequent visits.

The educator must be well-trained about asthma management. Adequate asthma education has been well documented to be poor in physicians, nurses, pharmacists, and respiratory therapists. Because of the increase in concern about asthma and the recognition that the presence of an educator may serve as a marketing device, the presence of self-proclaimed asthma educators of uncertain training has grown. Moreover, although the presence of published guidelines for asthma management are beneficial, they do not suffice for training an asthma educator. The American Lung Association and other groups now advocate licensing asthma educators.

Educational Techniques

A variety of educational techniques can be used to teach asthma management. Different patients may learn best with different techniques and, thus, a variety of techniques, such as those as listed in Table 9.2 should be used.

Pertinent Subjects

The topics covered in teaching sessions may vary depending on the forum. For example, during an emergency room visit, the concept of early warning signals leading to an impending asthma attack can be reinforced. However, the patient may be too overwhelmed to absorb an organized lesson in environmental control. During an inpatient stay, when there is more time available for teaching, more detail on medications and their use might be covered. In the ambulatory setting, where multiple sessions might be given, information on chronic management, including recognition and avoidance of triggers, might be more pertinent.

Simple Concepts/Limited Material

It is important to gauge the amount of information that a patient will be able to absorb and retain during a session. One approach stresses the use of individual issue-focused concepts. At each visit, only a few concepts are taught and reviewed. They should be pertinent to the patient's problems. Thus one visit of a patient with recurrent symptoms may be devoted to the recognition of triggers such as cleaning. The patient and family will then be taught techniques to clean the house which minimize the risk for an asthma exacerbation. Simplified educational material which supports each individual concept can be provided to reinforce the verbal education the patient has received.

Skills-Oriented Teaching

Retention of information is improved if the patient participates in the learning process. This participation also will demonstrate to the educator that the information is being transmitted. Interactive sessions can use specific material designed to allow the patient to answer questions. The "Asthma I.Q.," developed by the National Heart Lung and Blood Institute, is one such example. Patients should be requested to recall or demonstrate their own medications to the provider, rather than have the provider list them. Often this will reveal confusion and allow the educator to address hidden problems. The proper administration of medications via metered dose inhalers or spacer devices and peak flow monitoring are critical to asthma management. In addition to didactic teaching, education about asthma must incorporate skills teaching in these areas. The educator should demonstrate technique on a one-to-one basis, and the patient should then do a repeat demonstration. Visual aids may be used as well. Active participation in the learning of skills enhances the patient's understanding and ability to adhere to a treatment regimen.

Repetitive Teaching

The number of topics covered and interest or receptivity level of the patient can influence the amount of information absorbed by the patient, and the patient may forget what has been described. Therefore, teaching protocols should include repetitive teaching. This may mean repeating the same lesson at a different time or having a different educator repeat the same material in a different context. For example, we supply large volume spacers in our clinic. The use of the spacer is reviewed repetitively by the nurse and physician during most visits and on every occasion for the renewal of the spacer.

Appropriateness of Teaching

Teaching should be both culture- and age-appropriate. This is particularly important for asthma, where morbidity and mortality are most prevalent in predominantly African-American and Hispanic inner-city populations. Educational sessions and material should be presented in the context of the patient's social environment and in the patient's language of choice. Difficulties in translating educational material are made even greater by the presence of multiple dialects in many languages. Literacy may also be minimal.

Educational Tools and Written Materials

Information can be presented in multiple formats, including face-to-face individual sessions and small group sessions. Both formats have been demonstrated to be successful, and their success may depend both on the individual patient and on the educational program (Wilson, 1998).

There is an abundance of written material available for a variety of target audiences; quality is variable. When using written material, it should be matched to its use and target audience (Bauman, 1997). Some material may be developed for use on its own. Pamphlets and brochures containing extensive information may be useful for motivated, literate patients who will read them. Many of these materials are available from the National Asthma Education Program, NIH, or the American Lung Association. For more focused teaching, single-concept written material can be used to reinforce topics. This material should be appropriate for the reading level of the target audience and, ideally, should be used to reinforce the verbal advice. In our clinic, we have developed single concept, bilingual (English and Spanish) written material that has been literacy-tested at a 4th-grade level. This material is used to reinforce training sessions in the clinic, emergency department, and hospital. Although invaluable in these situations, the material would not stand alone. Comic books and workbooks are also available. Many of these, such as the "Asthma I.Q.," require patient interaction and are often fun for the patient. They may be very helpful for educating the child as well as adults. Finally, written material should be used when the patient has reached the level of self-management. This material should include written plans for chronic management, as well as for the management of an acute episode. Examples which can be tailored to the patient and his or her needs are supplied in the NAEPP guidelines.

Additional educational material increasingly is being made available on videotape. These, too, can be obtained through the NIH or the American Lung Association. All educational materials should be reviewed for accuracy as well as for age, language, and cultural appropriateness. Computerized programs or games are now being developed and may provide an exciting alternative way to reinforce educational material. However, their use will be limited to those who have access to computers.

A personalized written self-management plan is a long-term goal of many patients. Plans for daily management in which a patient may be instructed to change medications based on symptom and peak flow measurements can be developed. A different written plan may need to be developed for the management of an acute exacerbation.

In summary, asthma is a difficult disease for patients and their families to understand and accept because of the chronicity and variability of the disease. Techniques used to provide information should take advantage of "teachable moments" as well as multiple teaching techniques; they should be skills-oriented, and they should be repeated continuously.

Teaching Algorithm

A logical approach to management consists of teaching about recognition and avoidance of triggers, pharmacologic management, delivery of medications, and self-management techniques.However, this sequence usually is not feasible when treating a patient. For example, although the avoidance of triggers is the first line of therapy, this may not be the first issue discussed at the initial visit, when it often is necessary to stabilize a patient medically. In this situation, teaching is more effectively focused on the immediate needs of the patient; i.e., the appropriate use of prescribed medications. The identification and avoidance of specific triggers should be discussed during subsequent visits.

Our stepwise approach to educating patients with asthma in our clinic appears below. The teaching is based on the NAEPP guidelines but modified for use in our program. An algorithm of topics and their sequence for teaching in the ambulatory setting is proposed in Table 9.3.

Table 9.3   Bellevue Hospital Primary Care Asthma Clinic Teaching Algorithm

Topics	Initial teacher
Visit 1 (duration 1 hour)	
1. Basic concepts of asthma Inflammation in the airway Smooth muscle contraction Mucus production	Provider reinforced by nurse/educator
2. Role of pharmacologic agents a) Medicines to *prevent* asthma/in- flammation inhaled steroids or cromolyn + long acting β_2 agonist or theoph- ylline, LT modifier b) Medicines for *quick relief* relax muscles -β_2 agonists	Provider reinforced by nurse/educator
3. Medicine delivery techniques (verbal and skills demonstration) a) Review use of metered dose inhaler b) Review use of large volume spacer	Nurse/respiratory therapist/provider
4. Presence of "Hotline" Importance of alerting provider to changes in symptoms	Provider/nurse/respiratory therapist

Table 9.3 *(continued)*

	Topics	Initial teacher
Visit 2 (within 2 weeks of initial visit, duration 1 hr)		
1.	Asthma triggers Identify triggers/environmental issues and discuss specific trigger avoidance	Provider reinforced by nurse/educator/group
2.	Review pharmacologic agents and adjust a) Medicines to *prevent* asthma/inflammation b) Medicines for *quick relief*	Provider reinforced by nurse/educator
3.	Review medicine delivery techniques a) Review use of MDI b) Review use of spacer	Nurse/educator Respiratory therapist
4.	Begin Basics of self-management—monitoring asthma a) Recognition of early warning signals for asthma b) Use of peak flow meter Skills demonstration Start patient on daily peak flow chart for baseline monitoring	Provider/nurse educator Provider/nurse educator/respiratory therapist
5.	Identify obstacles and concerns	Provider/nurse educator, respiratory therapist

(continued)

Table 9.3   *(continued)*

Topics	Initial teacher
Visit 3 (approximately 1 month later, duration 0.5–1 hr)	

1. Review pharmacologic agents and adjust
  a) Medicines to *pre-vent* asthma/ inflammation
  b) Medicines for *quick relief*
	Provider reinforced by nurse/educator

2. Review medication delivery techniques
  a) Review use of MDI
  b) review use of spacer
	Nurse/educator
	Respiratory therapist

3. Basics of self-management—review monitoring asthma
  a) Recognition of early warning signals for asthma
  b) Use of peak flow meter skills demonstration
	Provider/nurse educator
	
	Provider/nurse educator

4. Basics of self-management—written management plan based on early warning signals and peak flow chart, develop written self-management plan at appropriate level for patient	Provider/reinforced by nurse/educator
5. Identify obstacles and concerns	Provider/nurse educator, respiratory therapist
Subsequent Visits (spacing depends on individual, duration 0.5 hr)	
All topics reviewed repeatedly, with specific topics reviewed at different sessions	

Visit 1

1. Basic Concepts of Asthma

To enhance the understanding of why specific medications are required, patients and their families must learn basic pathophysiology of asthma. We focus on three simple pathophysiologic concepts: (1) airway inflammation and edema; (2) smooth muscle contraction; and (3) mucus production. The mechanism by which these three processes lead to narrowing of the airway and prevent air from flowing is explained with a simple diagram. The symptoms that the patient recognizes when this happens are reviewed briefly to place the physiologic process in a recognizable context.

2. Role of Pharmacologic Agents

Pharmacologic agents are introduced to the patient in a stepwise approach depending on the severity of the disease. The terms that are suggested by the NAEPP guidelines to enhance understanding of the use of these agents are "long-term control" and "quick relief" agents. The naming of medicines in this fashion may depend on one's teaching style. We have used these terms extensively for our education protocols and have found them helpful although we have also reinforced the use of the term "Preventer" for long-term-control agents to underline the role of agents in prophylactic use. In general, only medications that are being prescribed are explained to the patient.

Medications to Prevent or Control Asthma
Anti-inflammatory agents
Inhaled Corticosteroids
The current NAEPP guidelines recommend administration of an anti-inflammatory medication for any patient with persistent asthma.

What to teach.   Despite the central role of inhaled steroids in the treatment of asthma, patient adherence with these agents is often poor because they do not provide immediate relief. For this reason, the concept of airway inflammation and disease prevention should be stressed at the initial patient encounter. Their use as "preventer" or "controller" agents needs to be stressed repeatedly. Patients should be forewarned that symptoms will not resolve immediately with the use of these compounds but that after 1–2 weeks, they will notice an improvement. The dose of inhaled corticosteroid will vary among patients and will require continuous adjustment for individual patients. This too makes adherence more difficult. Simplified regimens enhance adherence, thus twice- and even possibly once-daily dosing may be preferred (Barnes, 1995). Because consistency in the use of inhaled corticosteroids also enhances adherence, a dose of inhaled corticosteroid should be maintained even when a patient is receiving oral corticosteroids.

Most patients are concerned about side effects of corticosteroids, and these are issues that should be addressed early. The more favorable benefit/ risk ratio for inhaled corticosteroids compared to oral should be stressed. The most common complication of inhaled corticosteroids is oropharyngeal candidiasis. Less commonly, patients may develop dysphonia or cough. The incidence of these side effects can be greatly reduced by the use of a spacer device, which should be provided and its use taught when inhaled corticosteroids are introduced. The use of this device has to be emphasized continuously. Mouth washing after inhalation also can reduce the incidence of these complications. The risk for systemic side effects depends on the dose, bioavailability, and metabolism of the drug. Possible systemic effects of thinning of the skin, adrenal suppression, increased bone resorption, and growth delay should be reduced with the use of the lowest tolerable dose after the patient has been stabilized (Barnes, 1995). The minimal side effects with lower doses should be stressed to the patient.

Oral corticosteroids

What to teach.   Patients should be taught to begin oral corticosteroids as "rescue" therapy early in the development of an asthma exacerbation. Some, but not all patients, can be supplied with a dose of oral corticosteroids to keep at home for this use. When a patient is proficient at self-management, he or she can be taught to begin a prescribed dose of this drug at the onset of well-defined early warning signals. Patients who begin the drug should notify their health care provider. It should be stressed to the patient that the early therapy with oral corticosteroids may reduce the duration of treatment, and thus the risk of side effects. However, self-management in which patients rely on boluses of oral corticosteroids because of their ease of administration should be strongly discouraged. The side effects of oral corticosteroids are great, and they need to be discussed extensively with patients.

Sodium cromoglycate, Nedocromil sodium

What to teach.   Because of the absence of an immediate effect, compliance with these medications may be difficult to obtain. Thus when teaching a patient about using sodium cromoglycate or nedocromil sodium, it is necessary to stress that these medications are preventive and that their effects will not be felt immediately. However, neither of these drugs have significant side effects, making them particularly useful in children.

Long acting inhaled beta$_2$-agonists

What to teach. When providing a long acting beta$_2$-agonist to patients, it is imperative that a clear distinction between different functions of the short- and long-acting beta$_2$-agonists be made. It should be emphasized that long-acting beta$_2$-agonists prevent/control symptoms, whereas the short-acting beta$_2$-agonists provide rapid relief of symptoms. It is strongly suggested as a way of reducing its potential for misuse, the long-acting beta$_2$-agonist be kept at home and not carried around. In addition, the long-acting beta$_2$-agonist is to be used twice daily only, whereas the short-acting beta$_2$-agonist can be used on an "as needed" basis.

Sustained release theophylline

What to teach. Although they sometimes are used as adjunctive therapy, theophyllines are no longer recommended as first-line therapy; however, their place in the armamentarium of asthma treatment varies. When teaching a patient about the use of theophyllines, it is very important to stress their role as preventive therapy rather than as a therapy for rapid relief. A common misconception among patients is the presumption that since theophyllines are oral medications, they are "real" medicines compared to the MDIs, and thus may be the only important one with which to be compliant. The patient should also be warned repeatedly not to take extra doses of theophylline for the relief of symptoms, or to use them on an "as needed" basis. Patients should also be alerted to notify their doctor if they start taking new medications, since many of these may alter the theophylline metabolism.

Medications for Quick Relief
Short acting beta$_2$-agonists

What to teach. It is important to stress to patients that the predominant effect of these medications is to provide "Quick Relief," but that the underlying disease is not affected and thus they should not replace the use of the "Controller/Preventer" medicine. Because of questions of tolerance and toxicity, current guidelines recommend that patients be advised to use these medications on an "as needed" schedule. When used this way, monitoring the use of the beta$_2$-agonists also allows one to assess changes in a patient's disease severity by determining the frequency of its use. Patients should keep records of their use of the beta$_2$-agonist. It should be explained that the need for more frequent dosing of beta$_2$-agonists is an Early Warning Signal of worsening asthma, and that additional long-term control agents are needed. Patients should be counseled about the possible dangers of overuse of beta$_2$-agonists.

Because these drugs are marketed under different brand names with a multitude of generic agents now available, each with a different appearance, it can become confusing to teach patients to distinguish among them. Most patients identify them by color, but because of the changes in pharmacy supplies, or perhaps in institutional formularies which may substitute equivalent brands, it becomes important to explain to a patient the generic chemical name, as opposed to a specific brand name. It is critical that patients bring in the exact MDI that they are using to confirm and to demonstrate its use.

3. Delivery of Medications

Use of metered dose inhaler (MDI)

Studies have repeatedly demonstrated that most patients, regardless of socioeconomic class, age, or gender, fail to use these devices correctly (McFadden, 1995). This problem is compounded by the fact that many physicians, nurses, and pharmacists do not know how to assemble or use MDIs correctly (Guidry et al., 1992). Faulty technique results in significant underdosing. The most common errors are in the coordination of the actuation with inhalation, inspiratory flow rates that are too rapid, failure to hold the breath after inhalation, and inadequate shaking of the medication before use. Occasionally, patients fail to remove the caps of their MDI. In addition, patients often have the misconception that MDIs are not "real" medicine, or that all MDIs are the same. Thus their compliance is reduced, and they become confused over their medications. Another problem with the use of MDIs lies in the failure of a patient to recognize that the medication canister is empty.

What to teach. The correct use of the MDI must be emphasized in the management of a patient with asthma. Correct teaching of MDI use involves active demonstration by a health care provider, demonstration of proper technique by the patient, and reinforcement with simple written directions. Regardless, patients often forget what they have been taught, and revert to the incorrect technique or develop new errors. Technique also may be inconsistent, especially when a patient is anxious during an exacerbation. These problems necessitate repeated review of the use of the MDI. The technique for currently available MDIs is described in Table 9.4. These directions are for the "open mouth" technique. Patients who are unable to coordinate the "open mouth" technique can be directed to use the "closed mouth" technique where the lips are placed directly on the MDI. The key points to stress are slow inhalation and breath holding.

These instructions hold for the metered dose inhalers that currently are on the market. However, a new group of non-chlorofluorocarbon devices are being developed, and they soon will replace these current pumps. Many of these new MDIs contain dry powder formulations, and their use will differ significantly. An initial example is budesonide, which requires placement in the mouth and rapid inspiration. Thus teaching of these devices will soon become even more complicated.

Use of spacer devices

Although in most studies, optimal use of the MDI results in the equivalent delivery of drug compared to a spacer, the poor technique demonstrated by most patients suggests that spacer devices should be used by most patients.

A number of spacer devices are available on the market. Each of these differ in the technique used for their actuation. In addition, the fine particle dose presented to the lung differs among the different spacer devices and depends on the MDI drug preparation (Schultz, 1995). The ease with which teaching can be performed varies with the different spacers. Thus the particular spacer device used for a patient depends both on the drug

---

Table 9.4   Proper Use of the Metered Dose Inhaler (Pump)

1. Remove the cap and shake the pump.
2. Hold the pump upright, 2 finger breadths away from your open mouth.
3. Press down on the pump once.
4. BREATHE IN SLOWLY through your open mouth as you count to 10.
5. HOLD YOUR BREATH and count to 10.
6. Breathe out slowly.
7. Do this again as many times as directed by your doctor.
8. After using the pump, always replace the cap.

being used and on the patient; however, for consistency, each patient should have only one type of spacer device.

What to teach.   Key points for the use of most spacer devices include stressing that patients inhale slowly, hold their breath, and actuate their pumps once for each breath. Cleaning of the spacer also must be taught. In a manner similar to teaching use of the MDI, patient education about spacer use requires continued reinforcement about the importance of the correct delivery of medicine. Spacer technique must be demonstrated to the patient and correct use by the patient displayed. Relevant simplified written material should be given as reinforcement. Finally, review of spacer use should be performed on repeated visits.

Many patients are embarrassed to use the spacer in public. If counseling fails to reduce this embarrassment, it is recommended that the patient use the spacer for all medications taken at home, particularly corticosteroids. The patient then requires repeated teaching in both MDI and spacer technique.

Use of nebulizers

What to teach.   Because of their ease of use, nebulizers are well liked by patients. Patients should be taught that correct use of spacer devices also provides equivalent therapy. Those for whom nebulizers are felt to be necessary should be appropriately trained. This includes warning them against preparing the medication for use in the nebulizer in advance, because the beta$_2$-agonists oxidize rapidly. Patients should be taught how to clean their nebulizers and when to cease their use and seek further help.

5. *Ready Access to Information*

Despite repeated educational efforts, patients may forget or be confused about concepts reviewed during the session. Moreover, they may later think of important questions, or may not know how to manage particular situations that have occurred at home. In addition, changes in asthma symptoms may develop. It is important that an arrangement be made whereby the patient can contact a health care provider to ask questions. Access to a "hotline" or on-call physician should be explained. The availability of this contact further strengthens the partnership development between the patient and provider.

Visit 2

1. Recognition and Avoidance of Triggers

The identification of specific triggers or allergens should be attempted in all patients (Hoover & Platts-Mills, 1995). Although a multitude of triggers and environmental stimuli may be recognized, not all of them may be conducive to interventions. A variety of triggers, including allergens, viruses, and chemical irritants, have been described. Some of these triggers are more prevalent in specific areas. For example, house dust mite allergens are abundant in humid areas but are almost nonexistent in areas of high altitude.

Common Indoor allergens

Indoor allergens often play a large role in precipitating asthma symptoms, and patients should recognize the potential indoor allergens in their homes, particularly the ones to which they can reduce their exposure. These allergens include those from household pets such as cats, dogs, and rodents. Cats are potent sensitizers and the allergen, *fel d* 1 is found in the cat pelt, saliva, and urine. In some studies, more than 30% of patients admitted to the emergency room for asthma exacerbations were sensitive to cats. An allergen from dogs also has been isolated and can be found in the saliva as well as the pelt. Rodents are a particular problem. Many children or schools have rodents such as gerbils, hamsters, mice, or rats as pets; mice and rats are quite prevalent in inner-city areas. Allergy to these animals is frequent. There also is a large role for house dust mite allergens. Two common species include *Dermatophagoides pternoyssinus*, which is more common in damp environments, and *Dermatophagoides farinae*, which is found in drier areas. These mites feed on human epithelium and can be found in floors, carpets, mattresses, and soft furnishings as well as soft toys. In some regions, sensitivity to cockroach allergen may pose a particular problem and in some areas, this sensitivity is more common than that to house dust mite. The American and German species of cockroaches (*Periplaneta americana, Blatella germanica*) are the most common. Infestation with cockroaches is extremely common, again particularly in the inner city, where high sensitivity rates are seen (Rosenstreich et al., 1997).

What to teach. Removal of the pet animal is the first line of treatment in patients with asthma who are sensitive to animals. The decision to remove a pet often involves the family and compliance with this request succeeds only when the family is aware of the severity of the patient's illness. Patients must be warned that they may not note an immediate improvement in symptoms because the allergen collects in house dust. After removal of the animal, patients should be advised to damp-mop their houses. Vacuuming to rid the house of residual allergen should be done by someone other than the patient. After vacuuming, the patient should remain absent from the room while the dust settles. Despite this, animal allergen may take months to be completely removed. Should the animal remain in the patient's abode, it should not be allowed in the patient's room, and nonallergic individuals should clean the house. Some studies have recommended that the cat be washed weekly to decrease the allergen load (Hoover & Platts-Mills, 1995). Patients also may need to be counseled about techniques to decrease rodent infestation. Schools should be counselled against pets which induce allergies, and children should be provided with other pets, such as fish.

Patients in whom allergy to house dust mite is suspected (presence of nocturnal asthma, positive skin test, specific IgE or recalcitrant asthma) should be taught to remove as much of the carpets or upholstered furniture as possible. Bedding and soft toys should be washed in extremely hot water (55°C) weekly. The suggestion also has been made that freezing soft toys rather than washing them may rid them of the mites without destroying the toy. Special plastic mattress covers with enclosed zippers also may be used. The efficacy and safety of acarisides (benzyl benzoate, pyrethoids, pirimiphos methyl and liquid nitrogen) remains to be determined.

Cockroaches are extremely difficult to eliminate. It is recommended that patients clean breeding areas. These include regions under stoves, under refrigerators, and in kitchen cabinets. The use of bait stations or boric acid rather than insecticide sprays is advised. Although it may be difficult to rid an apartment of cockroaches if a building is infested, the local load of allergen may be reduced.

Although dehumidifiers and air conditioners can reduce mold and bacteria loads, they may become contaminated with fungi. Therefore their use may not be advisable.

Common outdoor allergens

What to teach.   In extreme cases, and particularly on days of high pollen counts, patients can be advised to remain indoors with their windows closed. The use of an air conditioner or a HEPA (high efficiency particulate air) filter may reduce the indoor collection of pollen.

Drug and Food additives

What to teach. Sensitivity to ASA should be elicited and medications that may contain them should be identified. Patients should be advised to avoid all aspirin (ASA) (brand names reviewed). The nonsteroidal anti-inflammatory drugs (NSAIDs) that are available as over-the-counter drugs should be reviewed. Some food additives, including some preservatives, sulfites, monosodium glutamate, and food colorings, also have a recognized role in sensitivity.

Viral infections

There is a clear association between some respiratory viruses and the exacerbation of an asthma attack.

What to teach. Although exposure to respiratory viruses is not preventable, it can be recommended that patients avoid obvious exposure if possible. In addition, they should receive influenza vaccine annually. If patients are aware that upper respiratory tract infections trigger their asthma, they can be taught to change their treatment during the initial signs of an upper respiratory infection.

Exercise and cold air

What to teach. Inhalation of cold air also may be a trigger, and winter may be a difficult time for many patients. Patients should be encouraged to continue exercising. If exercise is a recognized trigger, a warm-up period and the use of premedication may enable continued activity. If necessary, the type of exercise may be changed. Cold weather may exacerbate bronchospasm, and on frigid days, patients should remain indoors or wear loose scarves over their faces to warm the inhaled air. The efficacy of these recommendations however, remains unproven.

Perimenstrual asthma

What to teach. The presence of this trigger may be elicited by a history of recurrent increase in symptoms before or during menstruation. A daily diary with peak flow measurements may help document these symptoms. The recognition of this syndrome may allow for self-management with early preventive changes in pharmacotherapy.

Emotional stress It is important to stress that although emotional stress may trigger an exacerbation of asthma by an unknown mechanism such as hyperventilation, asthma is not a psychological disease.

Pollution/Irritants/Occupation-related triggers

What to teach. The greatest source of indoor irritants is cigarette smoke, which contains more than 4,500 compounds, many of them respirable. Many of these compounds are likely to act as irritants and trigger bronchospasm.

The first step for a patient who is sensitive to indoor irritants to take is to remove the irritant. Cigarette smoking by the patient or by occupants of the patient's home should be strongly discouraged. Surprisingly, this recommendation is extraordinarily difficult for a patient to comply with. In our adult clinic, approximately 40% of the patients with asthma smoke! These patients need smoking cessation management along with their asthma management. Because it often is difficult for the patient to approach family members, they may need to be counseled by the provider. Further, the advice may carry more weight when given by a professional.

Select occupations can act both as sensitizers and triggers. These include those that involve molecules that may act as allergens (e.g., food processing, detergent manufacturing, laboratory animal workers, bakers) as well as those that may be due to organic chemicals (manufacturing, hospital workers, plastics industry). It is important to elicit a history of possible occupational triggers because treatment may then include removal of the patient from the offending agent, medications, and protective devices such as face masks. This history may be elicited by a diary or peak flow meter diary which may demonstrate a temporal pattern associated with airflow obstruction. Further testing may be required to demonstrate sensitivity.

Most investigators agree that elevated levels of pollutants in the air, including particulate matter, gaseous sulfur oxides and nitrogen oxides, and photochemical oxidants (ozone), may all act as triggers (American Thoracic Society, 1996). Sensitivity to air pollutants may be hard to elicit, but patients should be warned to remain indoors during days with elevated levels of pollution. Moreover, urban areas may have regions with higher levels of pollutants such as diesel exhaust because of an accumulation of diesel-fueled vehicles or airflow patterns (canyon effects). Patients can be counseled to avoid these areas if at all possible.

4. Self-Management

Skills for self-management. Self-management plans require two skills: the ability of a patient to monitor asthma symptoms, and the ability to alter behavior depending on the monitoring. We routinely begin a self-management plan by first teaching basics of monitoring and, depending on the ability of the patient, to master this skill and advance to individualized management plans.

Monitoring Asthma

Recognition of Early Warning Signals

Recognition of early warning signals and objective signs is critical for the patient. Studies investigating death from asthma consistently have identified the greatest contributing factor to be failure by both the patient and doctor to assess and appreciate the speed and severity of the onset of an attack, and thus delay treatment (Beasley et al., 1989). These early warning signals may include symptom changes, altered medicine use, or peak flow measurements as a simple objective parameter. The family as well as the patient should be taught the importance of recognizing early warning signals, as family members may be the first to recognize the changes in symptoms and signs.

Daily Diaries

Teaching recognition of early warning signals can start by reviewing symptoms that patients experience as an acute exacerbation of asthma develops. Early warning signals include:

- Increasing shortness of breath
- Increasing chest or back tightness
- Increasing cough
- Increasing frequency of daytime wheezing
- Increasing nocturnal arousals
- Increase in early morning wheezing
- Increased frequency of use of rescue beta$_2$-agonist

There are many methods to teach recognition of these signals. Having a patient recall the symptoms that led up to an attack often alerts him or her to specific signals. Prompting may be helpful, since many patients do not recognize specific symptoms as premonitions of an attack. These symptoms should then be stressed as early notification that airway obstruction is worsening. The events leading to that episode can be reviewed, and the patient may then recognize the early symptoms that might have been ignored.

Use of a daily diary is an alternative method. Many diaries have been devised, but it is important to remember that the simpler the tool, the easier it will be for the patient to use, and the greater adherence will be. Sometimes a simple checklist of symptoms is helpful. However, even if the patient becomes knowledgeable about early warning signals, the next step, getting him or her to act on that knowledge, is even more difficult.

Peak Flow Meter

Subjective symptoms often provide inadequate warning of an exacerbation of asthma. Many studies have demonstrated that there is much variation in the degree of breathlessness when compared to physiologic measurements of airflow obstruction (Clark et al., 1992). Some patients may have minimal symptoms, despite great airflow obstruction. Patients may have a blunted perception of dyspnea, or deny it altogether. Because of this discrepancy between clinical symptoms and airflow obstruction, the use of an objective measure of airflow is critical.

Peak flow meters are easy-to-use, portable monitors that measure the maximum rate of expiratory airflow following inspiration to total lung capacity. In the chronic management of asthma, the peak flow meter can provide valuable information for the physician, alert the patient to early detection of worsening asthma, and, in conjunction with a management plan, it can be used to define treatment decisions.

Readings have to be tailored to each patient. Published normal ranges exist; however, a patient with asthma may never reach normal readings, and therefore the use of serial readings from each patient optimizes the predictive use of the peak flow meter.

A major problem with the use of the peak flow meter is that the reading is effort-dependent. Therefore, reliable readings require good technique. Demonstration of correct use of the peak flow meter and patient skills demonstration is required for teaching. Simplified written reinforcement also is helpful. Documentation of the readings also is important. Many peak flow meters or daily asthma diaries come with charts for patients to graph their results. Whereas some patients are capable of this exercise, others are incapable of graphing. Alternatively, patients can be provided with a paper that combines a place for a simple daily diary as well as a column for notation of the peak flow reading, with the assumption that this is easier than graphing. When peak flow meters are first provided to patients, he or she can be asked to document daily readings to ascertain their baseline or "personal best." Ideally, these measurements should be performed twice each day, at approximately the same time, and before and after the use of the bronchodilator. This chart is then used to develop a management plan at a later visit.

Visit 3

4. Written Management Plan

A personalized self-management plan can be developed when a patient has begun to understand the importance of recognizing symptoms and measuring peak flow. A different written plan for the management of acute exacerbations may be required.

A common program uses color zones to alert the patient to worsening airflow. In this plan, the patient records his or her "personal best." A "green zone" is calculated to be 80–100% of the "personal best" and readings in this zone necessitate no change in therapy. A "yellow (caution) zone" is 50–80% of a patient's "personal best." Specific treatment changes are recommended when readings are in this range. A "red (danger) zone" consists of readings that are below 50% of the patient's "personal best." When readings are in this range, patients may be told to contact a physician or seek emergency treatment in addition to making changes in medication doses. There are in fact, peak flow meters available which have green, yellow, and red zones on them to reinforce this technique. An alternative technique is to make exact recommendations based on specific numbers. Again, the "personal best" is considered baseline, and readings below may require specific management strategies. Regardless of the technique that is chosen, the important concept is to provide the patient with clear, precise written instructions based on the measurements.

Changes in treatment that are recommended are personalized and medications are added or decreased in a stepwise fashion. Instructions may include the doubling of a dose of inhaled steroids for a moderate decrease in the peak flow. This may be followed by the addition of prednisone. Some patients already are on high doses of inhaled corticosteroids, and they might directly add oral corticosteroids.

The correct use of treatment plans based on peak flow measurements allows patients a degree of control over their disease and thus improved confidence and well-being. In addition, the recognition of improved readings after a change in therapy provides positive feedback to the patient. However, some patients may not be able to follow an action plan, or they may be insecure about altering their medications on their own. We reinforce calling their providers if patients have a change in symptoms or peak flow and has even the least doubt about the action to take. Despite the implementation of a self-management plan patients must have access to physicians and must be encouraged to call their physician when peak flow measurements are low, or if there are any questions. Self-management works only in the context of a continued patient-physician relationship.

5. *Identification of Obstacles and Concerns*

During each session, the patient needs to be questioned about problems with medications, environmental issues, and management. Questions should include inquiries into potential social, work, school, and family matters that may be impinging on asthma care. Issues in any of these areas may impact severely on a patient's willingness and ability to adhere to a management plan and need to be recognized and addressed when possible.

Additional Education Resources

A number of programs have been developed to educate families about the management of adult and childhood asthma. Materials, guidelines, and support networks are available. There are a large number of educational resources for patients on the market. All materials should be checked for race, age, and cultural appropriateness as well as for accuracy, before being recommended to patients.

For the professional, teaching manuals include "Open Airways" which was developed and extensively tested by the Columbia University Department of Pediatrics. Manuals for schools which include training in awareness, as well as management are also available.

A complete listing of many of these materials can be obtained from the
National Asthma Education Program
P.O. Box 30105
Bethesda, MD 20824-0105
Telephone: (301) 951-3260

Chapter 10
HIV Infection and AIDS

Rona Vail, Jay Laudato, Steve Albert, and
Elizabeth Joglar

Current Trends in HIV Epidemiology

Almost 20 years after the first cases of AIDS were diagnosed, HIV infection and AIDS continue in epidemic proportions in the United States. As of June 1998, there were 665,357 cumulative AIDS cases reported in the US, with 54,407 reported cases for the period from July 1997 through June 1998. From July 1997 through June 1998, adult men who have sex with men (MSM) continued to be the largest proportion of diagnosed AIDS cases (35%) and reported HIV infections (27%). During the same period injection drug users (IDU) accounted for 26% of AIDS cases and 17% of reported infections. MSM with injection drug use accounted for 4% of AIDS cases and 3% of HIV infections. Heterosexual contacts accounted for 13% of AIDS cases and 16% of HIV infections. There were 385 cases of AIDS and 295 cases of HIV infection reported in children under 13 years old. Approximately 90% of both AIDS cases and HIV infections in children are attributable to perinatal transmission ("HIV Increasing," 1998).

HIV infections are increasing in women and minorities. In 1996, reported HIV infections decreased by 3% in men while they increased by 3% in women. HIV infections decreased 3% in African Americans and 2% in Whites, but they increased 10% among Latinos. Among youth (13–24 years) 44% of reported HIV infections occurred in females, 63% in African Americans and 5% in Latinos; 26% were heterosexually acquired, 31% were among MSM, and 6% were attributable to IDU ("HIV Increasing," 1998).

With the advent of highly active antiretroviral therapy (HAART) regimens, deaths from AIDS began a decline in 1996 which continues to the present. The rate of new AIDS cases also has been decreasing due to these effective treatment regimens, but diagnoses of HIV infection have remained stable from January 1994 through June 1997 ("HIV Increasing," 1998). Accordingly, there is an increasing prevalence of persons living with HIV, and providers in primary care settings are more likely to encounter patients with HIV infection.

Prior to HAART, the development of prophylactic therapies and effective treatments for opportunistic infections began to shift the locus of care for HIV/AIDS from the inpatient to the primary care setting. The advent of HAART (combinations of antiviral medications that include newer agents that are highly active) has continued to shift the focus toward ambulatory care by effectively reducing viral burden, thereby delaying the onset of symptomatic disease and significantly decreasing the incidence of new opportunistic infections. Accordingly, the treatment of HIV infection and AIDS increasingly has come to be considered a chronic manageable condition with an ambulatory/primary care focus.

However, with new technologies and treatments continually being introduced, and the need for rigorous treatment adherence to avoid viral resistance, the need for specialized, multidisciplinary HIV/AIDS primary care programs that can engage and support HIV/AIDS patients has become increasingly important. Health, social, and cultural factors also have a significant impact on patient access to and engagement in care, and they must be integrated into the development of HIV primary care programs and providers' efforts to educate patients to become partners in their care.

Health and Social Factors Affecting HIV Patients
Access to Care and Engagement

Several factors have an impact on a patient's ability to access and engage in medical care. The incidence of substance abuse and issues pertaining to mental health and social factors present unique challenges for primary care providers (PCPs):

> In many communities practitioners will provide care for patients for whom substance abuse, mental illness, homelessness, child care, lack of medical

insurance, and poverty are of more immediate concern than their HIV infection (Gallant, 1999).

In addition, cultural belief systems and sexual orientation are areas that providers need to understand and explore. An accurate assessment and understanding of the effects of health, social, and cultural factors will facilitate the provider's ability to effectively engage patients in care and improve treatment adherence.

Substance Use

The second highest incidence of AIDS is found in people who use intravenous drugs. Crack cocaine and alcohol also are significant factors in the transmission of HIV disease due to the increased frequency of trading sex for drugs and/or money. The provision of HIV treatment to active substance users poses serious challenges to providers. These challenges include: difficulty in keeping medical appointments and problems with adherence to complex treatment regimens; potential side effects due to drug interactions; and assessment of patient-identified clinical complaints (e.g., fever, nausea) which may be masked or potentiated by substance use.

A report by HRSA on substance use and HIV stresses that "access to primary care, drug treatment and other needed services is crucial to reducing substance abuse and providing effective therapy to the patient" (HRSA, 1998, p. 8). The PCP needs to be familiar with issues related to substance use, including physical and social impacts, drug interactions, and therapeutic options. All patients should be screened for substance use and linked to appropriate community resources for drug treatment and/or harm reduction services.

Mental Health

Routine assessment of the mental health status of patients with HIV infection is a key issue in a provider's ability to engage patients in care:

> Studies conducted among a number of different HIV infected populations, including gay men, substance abusers, and heterosexual partners, have found that within these risk groups, individuals who were HIV positive were

more likely to have a diagnosable psychiatric illness prior to developing HIV infection (O'Dowd, p. 4).

PCPs need to develop comprehensive treatment plans that include referral for psychiatric evaluation when indicated. Providers should have knowledge of the interactions of psychopharmacological treatment and HAART. In addition, they should have access to internal supports and community resources for continued mental health intervention for patients. Access to these referral services will ensure that patients remain engaged in medical treatment.

Social Factors

The stigma of HIV/AIDS continues to present concerns among the groups that are most affected by the HIV epidemic (e.g., gay men, intravenous drug users, women, and minorities). These perceptions have impact on patients who may fear disclosure, breach of confidentiality, or a loss/lack of social supports if they seek HIV treatment.

Patients need to be reassured that HIV information pertaining to diagnosis and treatment is kept confidential. Providers need to identify mechanisms for access to community resources which increase social supports for patients and address issues of HIV care.

Patient Identity and Cultural Factors Affecting HIV Patients

Access to Care and Engagement

Gender

Women are a group with one of the fastest rising incidences of newly diagnosed HIV infections. They face numerous challenges in coping with an HIV diagnosis and participating in care, and they may be reluctant to seek treatment due to potential domestic violence or a lack of child care arrangements. Often they are the primary caregivers in the home, which may result in a delay of their own entry into treatment until they are further along in the disease process. They have the dual responsibility of developing patient-provider relationships for children or partners who also may be HIV-infected. Women need to become engaged in care and offered additional opportunities for community supports.

Providers should obtain accurate family/household histories and ensure that women are well informed about access to care and current treatment options. Providers need to educate women about the importance of early intervention and treatment, and link them with appropriate services that will facilitate their engagement in care. PCPs should discuss reproductive options and be aware of up-to-date protocols for the prevention of perinatal transmission.

Sexual Orientation

Providers need to be aware of issues related to homophobia and its impact on access to medical care. Lesbians and gay men may avoid revealing their sexuality to a provider out of fear of rejection and hostility. It is important that providers assess their own responses to working with patients who are gay, and provide an atmosphere that allows gay patients to "come out." In addition it is important to understand the diversity that exists within the gay community. In evaluating gay men, clinicians must remember that not all of them have HIV disease, and that gay men are not all at equal risk for HIV infection (Lynch & Ferri, 1997).

Cultural Considerations/Cultural Competency

Cultural identity involves shared social connections related to group behaviors, beliefs and practices. These cultural factors also influence a patient's acceptance of treatment and receptivity to the provider. It is important that providers understand the influence of cultural considerations in treatment acceptance, and integrate cultural competency regarding ethnicity/racial background, sexuality, and gender issues into the primary care setting. The patient who is firmly bedded with his or her cultural history will be more inclined to engage in care with providers who convey acceptance of cultural differences and can incorporate alternative views of medical treatment into HIV treatment.

In summary, patients need to be educated about the benefits of engaging in treatment. PCPs should integrate health, social, and cultural concepts into comprehensive treatment planning and become sensitive to the needs of HIV patients who are entering managed care. PCPs need to develop a multidisciplinary approach that supports patient access and entry to medical services. They should use the initial and subsequent encounters to reinforce the patient-provider relationship and the importance of engagement in care.

Clinical Elements of HIV Primary Care

Care Models

HIV care provides an important example of the need for a biopsychosocial model in caring for people with chronic diseases. The complexity of medical and psychosocial issues involved in HIV illness requires a care model that is comprehensive, involving an interdisciplinary team functioning together to provide coordinated care. Care can best be provided when medical, nursing, social work, mental health, health education and nutrition professionals are working together to meet the diverse medical and social needs of the patient, and have the knowledge and skills required to provide appropriate care. It also requires close coordination with community-based AIDS service providers (e.g., housing, drug treatment programs, education, and social support services).

HIV Specialist as Primary Care Provider (PCP)

In the early years of the epidemic, when there was little to offer patients in regards to antiviral treatment, it was commonly felt that outpatient HIV care was part of the realm of the general primary care provider, at least until the patient developed symptomatic HIV disease or AIDS. The field of HIV primary medical care has become enormously dynamic in recent years with the advent of newer antiretrovirals, and new tests for monitoring treatment efficacy. It has become increasingly harder to stay current unless a provider is spending a significant amount of time in HIV care, and caring for a significant number of patients. Care standards change in a matter of weeks or months, and guidelines for care are often out of date by the time they are published.

HIV care has increasingly moved out of the realm of the generalist. It has been shown in studies that people with HIV fare better when they receive services from HIV-experienced providers. Kitahata et al. (1996) showed that survival rates are proportional to the level of provider experience. In recognition of this and of the increasing complexity of the field, consensus has emerged that patients should have access to HIV-experienced providers, and that health plans allow HIV specialists and HIV-experienced providers to be primary care providers for people with HIV. Health plans need to ensure a sufficient number of HIV specialists as PCPs and educate consumers about their options in choosing a PCP with HIV experience. It is important to note that HIV specialists do not need to be infectious disease trained, and in fact are often internists, family practitioners, and nurse practitioners. The essential ingredient is level of experience and ongoing training in HIV care.

Care Team Members

While medical expertise is an important aspect of HIV care, medical providers also need to bring a primary care approach to this specialty. Understanding pathophysiology of disease and treatment options will not lead to effective treatment unless providers also consider the psychosocial and mental health issues that have been previously mentioned as barriers to accessing and engaging in care, and provide care in the context of a team. Nurses who understand HIV disease processes and HIV treatments help to provide appropriate symptom assessments and treatment education. Social workers and case managers are critical for dealing with mental health, social, and substance use factors that affect a person's ability to engage in care. They also provide an important link to community-based services. Health educators can provide important risk-reduction education and treatment education and provide outreach and HIV prevention services. Peer educators, either on site or as part of a linked community-based service, can provide significant support and education, and can model ways of dealing with a chronic illness. They can be more effective than health professionals in helping patients engage in care. The role of peer educators in HIV care and education will be highlighted further on.

Comprehensive Primary Care and the Effects of Managed Care

Managed Care and HIV

When looking to manage care in the most cost-effective manner, programs may look to streamline teams and increase productivity in order to keep costs down. Health insurance companies may not cover the costs of services provided by some team members, or may try to limit formularies. These measures can adversely affect health outcomes and often end up costing more in the long run, as has been shown in the example of protease inhibitor therapy.

When protease inhibitors first became available in 1996, there was significant concern that the price tags attached to these medications were higher than the benefits that would be seen through their use. In response, some payers kept these drugs off their formularies. A number of cost-benefit analyses over the past 2 years have shown the shortsightedness of those policies. There has been a significant reduction in the cost of care since the introduction of protease inhibitors due to a dramatic drop in both the number of hospitalizations and the incidence of opportunistic infections, not to mention the enormous benefit to patients.

Interdisciplinary care teams may seem like a costly model for care, but this too must be put in the context of overall benefit of care. Productivity requirements may increase the number of visits, but can significantly compromise outcomes. Several examples demonstrate the importance of time and team to educate patients and coordinate care.

Early Intervention

While great advances have occurred in the treatment of HIV infection, the benefit clearly is the greatest when treatment is begun early in the course of HIV infection. Early intervention in the disease course can effectively delay or prevent progression to AIDS and death. In spite of this, many people are still entering into care with late-stage infection, sometimes first being diagnosed upon hospitalization for an opportunistic infection such as PCP pneumonia. Death from AIDS is still a significant reality, particularly when newer treatments are accessed late or not at all. Late entry into care is closely tied to the social and cultural barriers previously described.

Health education and community outreach that is culturally appropriate are important components of HIV programs and community-based AIDS organizations for bringing people into care, despite the multitude of barriers that keep them away. Effective community outreach can significantly decrease the costs of care and improve outcomes when it brings people into care earlier than would have otherwise occurred.

Once care is begun the challenge is to keep patients in care, and assist them in adhering to a treatment plan so that they can best attain the benefits of earlier intervention and preventive measures. This is best achieved by a comprehensive evaluation and treatment plan that encompasses the full spectrum of medical, mental health and social needs. The initial comprehensive evaluation includes:

- Detailed medical assessment including history, physical and laboratory parameters to appropriately evaluate the stage of HIV infection
- Mental health assessment
- Detailed social history including relationships, work, family, housing, social supports and coping skills, and assessment of substance use

A successful treatment plan must be based on the diverse aspects of the comprehensive evaluation and includes:

- Counseling on risk reduction and safer sex, partner notification
- Instituting appropriate prevention and prophylactic measures
- Determining an antiviral regimen and plan for monitoring and follow-up
- Mental health treatment plan
- Appropriate referrals as needed for housing, insurance and disability benefits, substance use treatment and harm reduction, support groups, etc.

Antiviral Therapy and Adherence Issues—Seizing the Teachable Moment

Determining an antiviral regimen provides a good example of the importance of considering all of the components of the comprehensive assessment in determining a treatment plan, and the potential pitfalls of narrowly focusing on medical data alone to prescribe antiviral therapies. To best illustrate this, some background information on adherence issues and HIV treatments may be helpful. Much has been written about treatment adherence, or the taking of medication in the amount prescribed at the appropriate intervals. Adherence issues are not new to HIV treatment, but HIV treatment poses interesting challenges for adherence.

There are a number of factors that influence the ability to adhere to a treatment regimen. Important considerations include the complexity of the regimen, the duration of treatment, the degree to which treatment interferes with daily life, side effects, belief in the effectiveness of treatment, and understanding of the reasons why adherence is important. Antiviral treatment poses significant challenges in these areas.

Antiretroviral regimens are complex. Guidelines presently advocate first-line treatment that includes a combination of two drugs known as nucleoside analogs (NAs) in combination with one or two protease inhibitor drugs (PIs). PIs can have significant side effects, have a high pill burden (6–20 pills in combination with NAs), and have food restrictions (some must be taken on an empty stomach, others with meals). In addition, PIs must be taken multiple times per day (2–3) on a rigid schedule as they are quickly cleared from the system. Skipping doses or taking doses later than scheduled leads to low drug levels and quickly leads to the development of viral drug resistance. Unfortunately resistance patterns for PIs have significant overlap or cross resistance, which means that development of resistance to one protease means development of partial or total resistance to the other PIs as well. The chronic nature of the treatment must also be taken into account, as patients must adhere to complex regimens in a perfect/near-perfect manner for years.

Recent studies have shown the degree to which adherence is a problem in antiviral regimens. In one survey of patients at clinical trial sites, 11% had skipped a dose of medication the preceding day, 14% had skipped a dose within the past 2 days, and 36% had skipped a dose within the past 2 weeks. Reasons given for skipping doses included: simply forgot (40%), asleep (37%), away from home (34%), change of routine (27%), busy with other things (22%), too sick (13%), side effects (10%), and depression (9%). Clearly, strategies for increasing adherence will need to address these issues as much as possible.

In determining who will have difficulty with adherence, there are some general correlations including younger age, active use of alcohol and drugs, stress, negative mentality toward treatment, and most significantly, depression. It is extremely important to note that these generalizations do not predict individual adherence and that each case must be taken individually. Studies have shown that patients who might be predicted to have poor adherence (homeless, active substance users) often have quite good success, and stability in life does not predict success.

Medical providers are unable to predict who will adhere to treatment. In a study presented at the 6th Conference on Antiretroviruses and Opportunistic Infections (Chicago, February 1999), Paterson et al. compared physicians' perceptions of patient adherence with reality (as determined by the use of MEMS caps). Twenty-one percent of patients who were predicted to be poor adherers were found to take > 95% of doses. Conversely, 29% of patients in whom providers predicted excellent adherence, took less than 80% of doses.

Choosing an Antiviral Regimen and Developing a Treatment Plan

Clinical Scenarios

Martha R. is a 29-year-old mother of two who recently learned of her positive HIV status after her daughter was found to be HIV+ at birth 3 months ago. She was referred to you by her daughter's pediatrician. She feels OK except for problems with fatigue and a poor appetite. Her physical exam is normal.

Plan

You recommend treatment based on a moderate degree of immune dysfunction as demonstrated by laboratory parameters including T cells and viral load. You recommend a three-drug combination regimen consistent with published treatment guidelines. After explaining the regimen including drug dosages and schedule, and potential side effects, you ask the patient to return for a repeat laboratory test in 3 weeks, and return in 1 month.

Discussion

While the clinician has followed appropriate treatment protocols, this treatment regimen has a significant risk of failure by not exploring potential barriers this patient may face in terms of adherence. The same clinical scenario using a comprehensive treatment plan to maximize adherence will now be discussed to compare and contrast strategies.

Plan

You determine that a three-drug combination regimen is clinically appropriate. However, you are concerned about how the patient is coping with the impact of this recent diagnosis, and are concerned that she may be depressed. You are also concerned about the tenuousness of her living situation. You decide to explore these concerns and have a social worker evaluate this patient prior to beginning treatment.

The social worker reports to you that while Ms. R has indeed gone through significant life changes, she has a good social network including a supportive family and friends, and does not appear to be clinically depressed at this time. She has made a referral to a patient support group and has recommended short-term supportive counseling. She has also begun the process of helping the patient to secure permanent housing and assistance with child care. You both decide that treatment initiation should wait one to 2 months while Ms. R gets services in place and begins supportive counseling.

Two months later, you and the patient agree that antiviral therapy is appropriate, and begin to discuss treatment options. You explore what factors are important to Ms. R in considering specific medications. You determine that while the number of pills is not an issue for her, it is important that the regimen not include pill-taking in the middle of the day if possible, because she is concerned that she will be busy with her kids or out of the house, and forget to take them. She can't eat a heavy breakfast in the morning because it makes her feel sick, and so needs medication that can be taken on an empty stomach, or otherwise with light meals. You develop a regimen that meets most of Ms. R's requirements. You now send her to the nurse for further in-depth review.

The nurse reviews the patient's understanding of the different medications, how to take them, and side effects. She then begins to review Ms. R's day, and helps her to strategize how to tie taking medications in with her daily activities, and how to balance mealtimes and pill times. They set up a schedule of times of day that Ms. R will take her medication. The nurse gives her a medication card that has her treatment plan with time of day and pills to take. She provides Ms. R with a pillbox, and recommends that she set the pills up for the week to serve as a reminder. She also gives her a medication alarm that will sound at the times that Ms. R will take her medications as an additional reminder. She asks Ms. R to return in a week so that she can review how things are going, and gives her phone number in case of any questions and concerns. She strongly recommends that Ms. R attend the treatment support group that is run at the clinic by peer counselors to help deal with medication issues. She introduces Ms. R to the peer educator, and informs her that child care is available during the group.

Another example of an individualized treatment plan and adherence strategy is the following:

Robert G. is a 32-year-old bookkeeper who comes to you to begin treatment for HIV. After an in-depth discussion you determine the following issues: he has difficulty swallowing pills and feels strongly that the less pills the better for him; and he lives at home and is not ready to reveal his HIV status to his family. He therefore can not take pills that need to be refrigerated, and he never eats breakfast. You devise a regimen that includes 3 drugs with a total of 8 pills, one of which must be taken three times a day on an empty stomach. The nurse sets up a schedule based on his daily routine and sets his watch alarm so that he does not forget to take his middle-of-the-day dose. The social worker recommends counseling to deal with revealing his HIV status as well as discussing his sexuality with his family, and refers him to the peer counselor.

Discussion

The above examples point to the need to develop a treatment plan that is comprehensive to best facilitate adherence. Successful adherence to antiviral regimens is critical to achieving long-term benefits from antiviral treatments. Health plans clearly benefit from the resulting decrease in morbidity and mortality that comes from effective antiviral use, and also suffer the consequences of nonadherence, resistance development, and disease progression. Investing in programs that are comprehensive and mutidisciplinary has costs in the short term that are more than outweighed by their benefits in the long term. Developing and supporting programs that maximize adherence has a positive impact on health plans, the individual patient, and public health.

Peer Education to Support Access and Adherence to Care

Over the last decade, peer education has become a central component of most well-designed HIV programs. With managed care driving today's health care delivery system, peer education can be a major contributor to minimizing the cost of health promotion. Peer education, simply defined as instruction or guidance from equals, delivers risk-reduction messages, treatment education, and supportive counseling to various target populations, while providing a service with an economy of cost (Gould & Lomax, 1993). Peer education, which is based on social learning theory, assumes that many people prefer peers, rather than professionals, to teach them about health issues. This assumption, which has crossed over into many targeted populations, is based on the fact that friends seek advice from friends, and are influenced by the expectations, attitudes, and behaviors of the groups to which they belong (Lindsey, 1997). Studies addressing attitude change and persuasion have shown that the credibility and similarity of the communicator to the person receiving the information can result in increased attitude change (Petty & Cacioppo, 1986). Peers have the power to influence behavior and attitudes, and to instill knowledge in people.

Peer education occurs in numerous forms. Programs nationwide implement health education interventions that take the form of one-on-one and group counseling as well as workshops, discussion groups, outreach activities, and case management. In addition, peers serve on advisory boards promoting health services, assist with quality assurance, staff outreach offices, hotlines, and health education resource centers (Sloane & Zimmer, 1993).

Integration into Outpatient HIV Clinic Setting

Peer education in outpatient HIV clinic settings focuses on secondary HIV prevention (prevention of disease progression and reinfection of the HIV positive patient). With all of the recent advances in HIV treatment and the reduction in both morbidity and mortality, the role of the peer educator has changed as well. Today, peer education interventions have HIV treatment education curricula at their core. Trained and experienced HIV-positive peer educators have developed counseling skills to provide support, to encourage treatment adherence, understand and manage side effects, and deal with the overall complexity of HIV medications. Peer educators also address such issues as re-entering the work world, taking control over one's life, and building self-esteem, as well as enhancing both sexual attitudes and negotiation skills.

In planning a peer education program, it is important to consider the numerous well-documented examples of peer education models nationwide. Health education professionals Beverlie Conant Sloane and Christine G. Zimmer remind program planners to build on the solid foundations that previous peer education coordinators already have laid (Gould & Lomax, 1993). All successful HIV peer education interventions have at their core, established comprehensive training curricula, multiple forms of supervision, and well-designed evaluation mechanisms. Peer education programs should be designed to respond to the needs of the target population. Peer educators serve as a bridge between patients and the health care system. Peer educators guide patients through a system, which often is perceived as a "scary world." A patient who is not comfortable disclosing information to a medical provider may feel more able to do so with a peer. The results of a well-designed peer education program will provide cost-effective benefits for the patient, and the team.

Benefits to the Patients

Speaking the language of the patient, peer educators empower patients to upgrade their involvement in their own health care. The empowerment of mirroring enables patients to take charge of their own health care. Peer educators encourage patients to ask more informed questions of their medical provider. This is especially important among those populations that feel like outsiders. By enhancing the traditional role of the social worker, peer educators can act as friends who help them tackle their fears of and concerns about the health care experience. Peer educators provide an emotionally safe space to ask shameful or embarrassing questions. Language and issues of the health care world are transformed into bite-size, digestible pieces.

Benefits to the Health Care Provider

In the climate of managed care, medical providers are being required to see more patients in less time. With little or no cost, peer educators can reinforce treatment plans and provide the supportive counseling necessary to allow providers to have more time to see more patients. They can provide additional support by enhancing the efforts of the medical provider. Peer educators can reinforce the treatment plans, medical messages, or educational agendas established by a medical provider. The health care provider also can learn from the peer educator about a patient's emotional or environmental condition and thus be more sensitive and, hopefully, more effective. Trained peer educators can identify patterns and trends of patients' issues or concerns that may aid the provider in better serving them.

Without a peer education component, the medical provider may be exposed to the patient only through the disease. Providers may gain personal insight by examining their own biases and prejudices that may exist regarding the target populations.

Peer educators also can benefit from this relationship. Recent studies have presented qualitative data that described changes in self-esteem, personal development, and sexual behavior among peer educators. Further research is needed that is aimed at improving the quality of peer education, and that looks at the effects that peer education has on the educator (Sawyer, Pinciaro, & Dedwell, 1997).

Securing Access to Care within a Managed Care Environment: Patient Education and Provider Advocacy

Providers should assist their patients who are enrolled in managed care plans to learn about their rights and options for securing needed care and services. In general, patients can obtain information about their rights and responsibilities through their health plan's Member Services office. Member Services offices distribute information to all enrollees about the scope of benefits covered by the plan and means of accessing services upon enrollment in the plan and notify colleagues whenever an update to these services or procedures occurs.

HIV primary care providers (PCPs) should acquaint themselves with the benefits and mechanisms for accessing care and services within the health plans in which they are participating providers. And, while patients must be educated about their rights and responsibilities and take an active role in accessing services within their managed care plan, providers' involvement usually is required to ensure that needed medical/clinical services are received. PCPs usually interact with the Utilization Management office of the plan in gaining access to needed services for their patients.

PCPs should be familiar with and assist their patients in gaining information on the following topics: all covered benefits and any limits on utilization; any required copayments or deductibles for services; appropriate means of arranging for a service (e.g., preauthorization by a provider); procedures for obtaining out of network services (i.e., needed specialty services from providers who do not participate in the health plan); policies on accessing emergency or urgent care services; policies on covering expenses considered investigational or experimental and any expenses associated with participation in a clinical trial or expanded access protocol; and procedures for filing a complaint/grievance.

Familiarity with the policies and procedures on these topics will help providers and patients to make the system work for them and thereby increase access and minimize any interruptions or breaks in needed services. Several of these issues are of significant importance to patients with HIV/AIDS and merit further discussion. These topics are: accessing out-of-network specialty services; accessing emergency and urgent care services; policies on covering expenses considered investigational or experimental and any expenses associated with participation in a clinical trial or expanded access protocol; and filing a formal complaint/grievance.

Accessing out-of-network specialty services is the most likely area where patients with HIV/AIDS will experience problems with their managed care insurance. Patients with HIV/AIDS can experience numerous clinical conditions or syndromes, many of which are specifically related to HIV infection, that require care by specialists who are experienced in HIV-related disease manifestations, particularly hematology/oncology, neurology, ophthalmology, dermatology, gastroenterology, and obstetrics and gynecology. Patients have the right to request information from their HMO about the training and experience of network providers. If it is determined that no provider within an HMO panel has specific experience in addressing an HIV-related condition, patients or their PCP can seek authorization to access the services of an out-of-network specialty provider or specialty care center. Different health plans have different mechanisms for approving out-of-network service. In general, however, patients can pursue this approval through the Member services office and providers through the Utilization Management office.

Although significant advances have been made in the clinical management of HIV disease, patients with HIV/AIDS are very likely to require emergency or urgent care services throughout the course of their illness. Patients and PCPs should be acquainted with what their specific health plan has established as covered emergency services as well as the procedure for obtaining authorization for these services. Usually, health plans operate a 24-hour telephone triage program that patients can use to get medical guidance on obtaining appropriate care for their problems and authorization for services. However, in most states, there are specific provisions that allow a patient to access emergency services without prior authorization under a "prudent lay person" standard. This standard means that prior authorization is not required if a patient with a general knowledge of health and medicine believes that he or she is experiencing an urgent health need "of such a nature that failure to obtain immediate medical care could result in (a) placing the patient's health in serious jeopardy; (b) serious impairment of bodily functions; or (c) serious dysfunction of any bodily organ or part" (Families USA Foundation). Providers should educate patients about this provision and inform them of what conditions, signs or symptoms warrant seeking immediate medical care.

Throughout the course of their illnesses, many patients with HIV/AIDS may elect to participate in clinical trials or expanded access programs. In general, no out-of-pocket expenses are incurred by patients or insurers in HIV/AIDS-related clinical trials. Most clinical trials also will cover the health care costs associated with adverse reactions attributable to the study therapy. However, clinical trials differ in whether they will cover the health care costs associated with adverse reactions attributable to the study therapy. PCPs and their patients should obtain specific information on this possibility as part of the informed consent process.

Expanded access programs generally fall into two categories: emergency use or compassionate release programs that make investigational new drugs available to patients who have failed standard therapies, and parallel track programs that make drugs that have completed safety testing available on a wide scale basis (AIDS Institute, 1995). In general, expanded access protocols do not cover the costs of care other than those of the expanded access drug. Costs of laboratory tests that are necessary to monitor patient responses to the therapy, needed complementary therapies (i.e., FDA-approved drugs used in combination), and adverse health results from use of the investigational drug are not generally included. Patients or their providers who seek to enroll in expanded access trials should ascertain these costs or potential risks through the informed consent process and determine if the plan will cover them.

PCPs also may seek to utilize therapies or procedures that are considered experimental or "off-label." Off label refers to the use of a drug for a purpose for which it has not been approved. For example, thalidomide, which was approved for the treatment of HIV-related wasting, recently has been used in the treatment of aphthous ulcers of the mouth and esophagus of patients with HIV/AIDS. In general, HMOs or other health insurers are reluctant to pay for investigational treatments or off-label drug use. Providers and patients who seek coverage for these treatments will have to pursue a formal process to gain coverage. This process generally can be initiated through the Member Services office or by the provider through the Utilization Review office of the plan.

A more widespread issue in caring for patients with HIV/AIDS has been timely coverage for newer diagnostic tests. Recent examples include coverage for newer generation laboratory assays that measure viral load (ultrasensitive HIV PCR) and new technologies that measure viral resistance to antiviral medications (genotypic and phenotypic resistance assays). While these tests are accepted as being important in clinical decision making on therapeutic regimens, these assays are not approved by the FDA and therefore may not be covered by insurers. In general, a request for coverage for a service that is applicable to all patients with HIV/AIDS can best be pursued by an HIV/AIDS advocacy organization. These organizations exist in most large metropolitan areas and there are several national organizations that can provide guidance and support on these issues for patients and providers. These groups include: the American Foundation for AIDS Research (AmFar), the AIDS Action Council, and the International Association of Physicians in AIDS Care.

Understanding the mechanism for filing a formal complaint/grievance is extremely important for both patients and providers. All health plans must develop and follow prescribed guidelines for receiving and deciding on formal complaints/grievances. In general, there are specific policies on making determinations on formal complaints based on the impact of the health of a patient. For example, complaints made that impact on continuing treatment such as an inpatient stay or home care services generally must be made within 24 hours. Pre-authorization for a service can take several days unless an expedited review is required due to a medical necessity. A dispute over a billed service or other nonmedically related service dispute can take up to a month or more for a determination.

The provider's involvement in a medical complaint is critical to obtain a clinically appropriate service. Providers also should familiarize themselves with community advocate organizations that can assist their patients in filing and obtaining decisions with regard to their complaints. Local AIDS service organizations or legal services groups generally provide this type of support to patients.

Chapter 11
Hemophilia*

*Susan Resnik, Shelby L. Dietrich, Regina B. Butler, and Craig A. Epson-Nelms***

Maximizing efficient and effective high quality care for hemophilia patients involves understanding both the combined scientific and clinical aspects of the disease and becoming knowledgeable about the social and cultural contexts within which they reside. In addition, familiarity with systems and ability to access resources developed by the well-organized, sophisticated national hemophilia community will provide a useful road map for providers and a ready-made support system for patients and families.

Hemophilia

Hemophilia is a genetic blood coagulation disorder secondary to a deficiency or absence of one of the plasma clotting factors either factor VIII (Hemophilia A) or factor IX (Hemophilia B) resulting in prolonged bleeding. All socioeconomic groups, races and ethnicities are affected.

*Many thanks to the following individuals for their input into or reviews of this chapter: Catherine Mintzer, Renee Paper, Glenn Pierce, Sarah Wiley, Sally Crudder, David Linney, and Richard Lipton.
**Deceased.

Editors' Note: Many might consider hemophilia an esoteric topic for a book such as ours. We have elected to include it because of the significant, excellent work in collaborative care, patient and family education, and peer education for a life-long, complex chronic disease.

The estimated incidence in the United States ranges from 1 in 5000 (Soucie, Evatt, & Jackson, 1998) to 1 in 7500 (Lusher & Warner, 1991) live male births. Factor VIII deficiency is about four times more common than Factor IX deficiency (Manno, 1991). Because the defective gene is on the X chromosome, a female carrier will have one abnormal X chromosome and one normal X chromosome. There is a 50% chance that each of her daughters will be a carrier and a 50% chance that each of her sons will have hemophilia. Since affected fathers have the affected gene on their only X chromosome, all of their daughters will be obligate carriers and all of their sons will be normal (Miller, 1991).

Bleeding can occur in any part of the body. Life-threatening episodes occur specifically in intracranial bleeding, airway obstruction (neck and throat edema), and gastrointestinal bleeding. These can occur with or without trauma and require immediate treatment and evaluation. Joint bleeding is the most common site; repetitive episodes usually progress to degenerative joint disease.

Accurate diagnosis in conjunction with an experienced hematologist, using a reputable coagulation laboratory, is essential. Obtaining a family history, including a family tree, is required. If either a suspected or known carrier is pregnant, genetic counseling is essential.

Bleeding in hemophilia is treated by replacing the deficient factor. Traditionally, factor replacement products have come from pooled human plasma. Since 1992, technology has allowed patients and families to choose a plasma-free recombinant product emanating from DNA technology. Currently available plasma products undergo screening and significant purification and viral inactivation. Concern for maximizing both safety and purity has driven the recent advances, producing improved safer products. Due to these techniques, no person with hemophilia has been infected with HIV through treatment products since 1987. Hepatitis C also has been virtually eradicated from the newer products. Prophylactic administration of concentrate in early childhood can prevent most secondary complications (Lusher, 1992). These advances have created the possibility of a normal life span and a normal lifestyle for young children and for older individuals who were not affected by HIV.

Von Willebrand Disease

Von Willebrand Disease (vWd) is the most common inherited bleeding disorder. It affects between 1% and 2% of the population and both sexes are at risk (Hoots, 1995). This condition is caused by a deficiency or defect of von Willebrand factor (vWF). It is manifested by easy bruising and mucous membrane bleeding such as nosebleeds, gastrointestinal bleeding, menorrhagia, and excessive bleeding following dental work and surgery.

Misdiagnosis of the condition occurs frequently when it is assumed that hormonal problems have caused dysfunctional uterine bleeding. A coagulation disorder is suspected only when menorrhagia becomes severe and intractable to conventional therapies, often when women are in their late teens or early twenties. Internists, obstetrician/gynecologists, and family practitioners should include vWd in their differential diagnosis of these patients.

The Hemophilia Treatment Center Network

There are 140 federally funded hemophilia treatment centers in the national HTC network. All HTCs have multidisciplinary teams of health care providers who collaborate in diagnosing and treating patients with hemophilia or von Willebrand's and their families. They develop and institute individualized treatment and educational plans and coordinate the complex range of medical and psychosocial services needed for each patient. The care teams usually consist of the patient/family, a hematologist who specializes in hemophilia and von Willebrand's, a nurse clinician/coordinator, a social worker, and a physical therapist. Other disciplines that usually are included are genetic counselors, psychologists, orthopedists, and gastroenterologists. Thus, the approach stresses comprehensiveness and continuity of care concerned with the total person within the context of his or her family and community.

The availability of factor concentrates, pooled plasma, new recombinant products, and introduction of self-infusion has enabled patients and families to treat most bleeding episodes at home, school or work, reducing absenteeism and minimizing disruption of the family's lifestyle.

Function of Comprehensive Care Centers

Comprehensive care centers have many functions, some of which change, over time, as advances in care, complications, and treatment issues arise and health care issues evolve, requiring adjustments and flexibility in services.

Diagnosis and Evaluation

Hematologists, experienced in coagulation, will perform testing to diagnose individuals with hemophilia, or vWF at the HTCs or in consultation with a local medical provider. Testing should be done in an HTC laboratory or in one with extensive coagulation experience. Once diagnosed, counseling and education are provided for the individual and his or her family.

Treatment

The HTC team assesses and treats acute bleeding episodes and coordinates care provided by community and other specialty providers.

Education

Education of the patient and family, community, and other medical providers about the unique needs of patients with hemophilia is one of the primary responsibilities of the comprehensive hemophilia team.

Patient and family education is a primary responsibility for the physicians, nurses, and social workers in the HTCs. It begins at the time of diagnosis and is a lifelong process for the parents, child, siblings, extended family members, and the older patient with hemophilia. The goals are to enable the parents of the individual with hemophilia to become active, informed participants in the total care of hemophilia and to promote independence and allow for sound decisions which promote optimal health. Informal and formal education sessions are scheduled to assess the learners' interests, knowledge, and needs, and to plan the individualized education program for each family or learner.

Hemophilia Treatment Center staff use a wide variety of materials to enhance their patient/family education efforts. Many are developed by the hemophilia provider groups with support from the National Hemophilia Foundation; many are prepared specifically for a group of patients by the HTC staff; and others are developed with grants from various agencies, including the pharmaceutical companies that manufacture factor concentrates.

Communication

During evaluations, staff spend time with the patient and family to review issues of concern to them, discuss progress and problems, and develop a plan of care. HTC staff are readily available to answer questions and help solve problems that arise between visits. Twenty-four-hour coverage for emergencies is provided. Staff maintain verbal and written communication between the HTC and the primary medical provider and other specialists involved in an individual's care, as well as school personnel, employers, insurance representatives and others, as requested by the family.

Comprehensive Clinic Evaluations

The frequency of comprehensive hemophilia evaluations vary from center to center. Core activities, however, are similar in every HTC. The team obtains a careful history of bleeding, treatment, and other medical issues, and answers questions. Physical assessment and laboratory studies, and any indicated x-rays are performed and interpreted, and joint function and muscle strength are assessed carefully. New trends in treatment and options for the individual are presented. Each patient and family participates in choosing factor replacement products and home delivery services. Usually, opportunity for peer interaction is offered. In all cases, problems are identified and providers and family members develop an ongoing plan to address identified issues.

Data Collection and Research

Data are often collected about numbers of bleeding episodes, hospital admissions, and laboratory tests such as hepatitis markers and inhibitor levels. All HTCs in the federal network collaborate with the Centers for Disease Control and Prevention (CDC) in collecting information and developing plans to prevent complications and promote optimal outcomes for patients with hemophilia. HTCs also provide access to protocols related to hemophilia hepatitis, HIV, inhibitors, and other complications of hemophilia. Newly diagnosed babies with factor VIII or factor IX deficiency have the opportunity to participate in trials of newer, potentially safer treatment products, through HTCs.

Summary

Documented cost effectiveness such as success in reducing the rate of hospital admissions and increasing the ability of patients to attend school and to be fully employed, motivated Congress to declare hemophilia "one of the bio-medical successes" of the decade in the late 1970s. Current studies reveal that over 20 years of experience in treating patients with this condition in a comprehensive manner has also resulted in lower death rates within the HTC network than outside of it (Soucie, 1998).

Alternative Models in the Managed Care Era

The changing health care delivery system undoubtedly will affect patients and families with hemophilia and vWd. Change is always difficult. In this case, it involves redefining roles for both providers and consumers. Reluctance to alter the existing situation has been expressed by both patients and providers. However, collaboration and communication are essential to help patients and families, as well as medical providers, adjust to evolving systems and maintain access to high-quality care. Comprehensive HTCs, the NHF and other providers, and consumer and government resources remain available for all individuals with inherited bleeding disorders. It is essential that none of the needed services for individuals with hemophilia fall "between the cracks" as a result of new medical care configurations.

Primary care providers, case managers, and HTC staff must continue to increase communication and work together to develop optimal care plans for diagnosis, evaluation, treatment, education, and product distribution for all patients with hemophilia and vWF. Letters, referrals, educational workshops, and ongoing verbal communication are essential to the success of hemophilia care. Recognition of the potential for serious ethical considerations supports the importance of maximizing collaboration.

Primary care providers and others in managed care situations can benefit from drawing upon the existing HTC structure and utilizing the expertise provided. The vast array of both person power and medical expertise can augment education and care provided in other settings. Appropriate referrals to HTCs also will be mutually beneficial. As previously noted, a variety of patterns can be forged to maximize provision of high-quality care for these patients and their families. Contractual arrangements might be considered. In order to maintain standards achieved by the comprehensive care model, providers should strive to provide or to acquire care that is family-centered, will minimize complications from bleeding and treatment, will reduce school and work absenteeism, and will minimize family lifestyle interruption.

At this time, a wide variety of hemophilia health care models or arrangements exist. Many leaders from the hemophilia community state that the best arrangement would be for HTCs to be designated as primary care providers. The successful track record of HTCs, and the wealth of expertise developed over the past 20 years by hemophilia treatment center care providers, underlies this stance. Expressed concern is that absent the HTC, care will be fragmented and that patients will be seen instead by inexperienced providers. Even if there is a hematologist, if he/she has only seen one or two patients with hemophilia in the past, there may be a loss in quality of care. HTC providers have familiarity with the expectations of educated adult patients and their families, many of whom present with both HIV infection, hepatitis, and hemophilia. There are also concerns about the lack of availability of products of choice through HMOs or community providers with less experience or fewer patients.

Another favored arrangement, particularly by medical directors of regional HTCs based in academic medical centers, is one in which the HTC is designated a "center of excellence" and included as such within the managed care organization's network. A modification of this configuration is an "out-of-network" arrangement for certain components such as special laboratory coagulation studies deemed essential. The key issue is to sustain access to high-quality care developed by the HTC network bypassing obstacles and network limitations.

One current arrangement in the New York area involves the managed care plan contracting with an expeditor of chronic diseases who furnishes case management specialists to plan and facilitate access to necessary care and treatment for all their hemophilia patients. In Wisconsin, the HTCs employ a financial specialist who advocates for and implements the best arrangements for hemophilia patients by working on a collaborative basis with medical services directors and coordinators of local managed care plans; for the most part, these are working satisfactorily.

An alternative model would be to include HTCs in the managed care provider's network of specialty providers. As noted, individuals with hemophilia are best served when hemophilia care is received in a comprehensive hemophilia treatment center. Evaluation, diagnosis, and management of this relatively rare disorder requires experience and specific knowledge in an ever-changing medical climate. In pediatric populations, most children receive primary care from their community pediatric provider. When this provider collaborates with the HTC, optimal, yet convenient care is the result. In this model, well child care, anticipatory guidance, nutritional teaching, safety, and preventive immunizations are usually best provided by the primary care provider (PCP). Diagnosis of an inherited bleeding disorder, evaluation of acute bleeding episodes, comprehensive care and hemophilia teaching are provided by the HTC staff.

Seizing the Teachable Moment

Whether the first educational encounter occurs within an HMO, PCP or an HTC, concerns for maximizing the effectiveness of the teachable moment are the same. Congruence among all messages presented by providers is essential. Thus, the "team" extends beyond the walls of the HTC, and it becomes important to record and share what has been taught as a component of treatment notes. As noted previously, health care providers must also become knowledgeable about the nature of the disease.

This is the traditional model of hemophilia care in most areas and works well when communication is maintained between the HTC and PCP. The level of participation by PCPs in managing hemophilia-related complications varies according to location and the interests of the PCP. A well-informed PCP is a valuable member of the HTC team. He/she can reinforce teaching, assist in evaluating acute bleeds, and obtain needed laboratory studies. This approach is successful when the local provider and the HTC staff discuss each incident and develop a plan of follow-up together. Utilization of electronic technology, such as email, can enhance this communication. Complications are more likely to arise if communication with the HTC is delayed or initiated only after unsuccessful treatment attempts.

The nurse coordinator usually is the pivotal member of the HTC team who is responsible for ensuring that patient and family education is incorporated into the management of the condition. The National Hemophilia Foundation Nursing Committee has assisted nurses in fulfilling this function by fostering the development, field testing, and distribution of a multidisciplinary curriculum guideline, *The Hemophilia Patient/Family Educational Model* (PF Model) (Levine & Resnik, 1981). These authors recognized that all members of the HTC team have an educational component of their roles and provide a flexible guideline for management of the condition in a modular interactive format.

This educational tool promotes an adult education approach to learning. Emphasis is placed upon an educational interchange. Including family members in the educational process enables them to identify and better understand how and when they can be supportive to the patient. Patients and families are taught to identify crises and to learn the necessary steps to resolve them. Hemophilia treatment center staff learn to listen to patients and families and to respond appropriately. The value of listening to the informed patient and family cannot be overemphasized.

In the 1980s the U.S. Maternal and Child Health Bureau provided additional support for enhancing providers' educational competencies by funding provider education sessions throughout the country. They were based upon maximizing the use of the *Patient/Family Educational Model.* Since the advent of HIV and AIDS, the Centers for Disease Control and Prevention (CDC) also has contributed to the educational component of hemophilia care by supporting and guiding the development of curriculum-based provider training sessions designed to enhance both HIV risk-reduction efforts and update hemophilia provider education (Butler, 1996).

Beginning with a Core Curriculum (Table 11.1), education should be tailored specifically to the learner's needs, learning preferences, and education goals and objectives. The Timeline (Table 11.2) and the Simulated Prospective Case Study describe a continuum of education and illustrate how an educational protocol can be adapted for different stages of development and levels of maturity.

Listening to patients and families, and attempting to see through their eyes and stand in their shoes, may be the best method of beginning an educational intervention. Educational priorities for individuals and families can be established within a framework of a patient/family partnership. Reality checks can enable providers to meet basic needs first, determine the existence of unanswered questions, dispel myths, especially family

Table 11.1 Core Curriculum: A Guideline to Hemophilia Education

Knowledge of	Competencies Skill in	Target Time Frame	Potential Learners (Patient/Family)	(Others)
Physiology of clotting	Understanding what hemophilia is	New diagnosis New relationship with person with bleeding disorder	Parents, grandparents, older siblings, extended family, babysitters	Home care nurses Day care providers Community medical providers
Diagnosis/Level of severity	Identifying diagnosis and severity of identified patient	New diagnosis New relationship with person with bleeding disorder	Parents, grandparents, older siblings, extended family, babysitters	Home care nurses Day care providers Community medical providers
Patterns of inheritance Basics of genetics Role of chromosomes X linked Carrier status/obligate carrier Prenatal diagnosis	Understanding risks of having an affected child; recognizing other individuals at risk Identifying genetic pattern on charts	New diagnosis Whenever sisters, other female relatives reach puberty or are considering reproductive options School age Courtship	Parents Pre-adolescents with hemophilia/von Willebrand Disease Sisters Extended maternal family members Potential partners	Obstetricians Community medical providers
Diagnosis: Recognition, laboratory studies types and severity	Recognizing warning signs of potential bleeding disorders; Understanding meaning of test results; Identifying severity and implications	New diagnosis Family planning Adolescence	Parents Adolescent patient Potential spouse/partners	Pediatricians Ob/Gyn

Table 11.1 *(continued)*

| | Competencies | | Potential Learners | |
Knowledge of	Skill in	Target Time Frame	(Patient/Family)	(Others)
Sites of bleeding/signs and symptoms	Recognizing most serious sites of bleeding; Recognizing need for early intervention	New diagnosis School age Begin/consider home treatment New relationship with person with bleeding disorder	Parents Grandparents Extended family Siblings Friends Potential partner/spouse	School staff School nurse Community medical provider Home care nurse Babysitters, employer
Prevention and safety	Identifying hazards; Providing safe environment	Infancy School age Adolescent Adulthood	Parents Extended family School age/adolescence children Friends	Hospital staff Pediatrician Home care nurse Day care center School nurse Phys ed/teacher Other school staff Coaches Community, etc.

(continued)

Table 11.1 (*continued*)

Knowledge of	Competencies Skill in	Target Time Frame	Potential Learners (Patient/Family)	(Others)
Signs and symptoms of bleeding	Recognizing early signs of bleeding; Assessing bleeding episodes	All ages New relationships with person with bleeding disorder	Parents Pre-school, school age and adolescents Adults with bleeding disorders Friends Partners Spouses	Caretakers Community medical providers (dentist, doctors) School Nurse Employers Comp nurse, etc.
Management of bleeding episodes	Seeking/Providing appropriate treatment	All ages, especially new diagnosis and people with new relationships with person with bleeding disorder	Parents School-age child and older adult patient Significant other/Spouse Adult offspring	School/community Medical providers Employers Home care nurses Insurance company
Philosophy of factor replacement/types of treatment protocols	Understanding types of available products and treatment protocols; Choosing appropriate product; Choosing prophylaxis or "on demand" therapy	New diagnosis School age Onset of joint bleeding Adolescence Young adulthood New relationships/marriage	Parents Person with bleeding disorder Partner/Spouse	Insurance company Community medical providers Home care nurse School nurse Employer

Table 11.1 *(continued)*

Knowledge of	Competencies Skill in	Target Time Frame	Potential Learners (Patient/Family)	(Others)
Appropriate physical activity	Identifying best activities for individual avoiding high-risk activities; Promoting physical fitness	Toddlers School age Adolescence Adulthood	Parents Siblings Grandparents Extended family Babysitters Friends Partners/spouses	*School* Nurse Phys ed teacher Teacher Recess aide Other Community medical provider Coaches Employer

(continued)

Table 11.1 *(continued)*

	Competencies		
Knowledge of	Skill in	Target Time Frame	Potential Learners
			(Patient/Family) (Others)
Psychosocial implications	Recognizing psychoso-cial, cultural and finan-cial issues which impact families;	New diagnosis	Parents
Adaptation to illness		Recognition of "differences"	School age children and adolescents
Reaction to diagnosis		New school	Adults with bleeding disorders
Financial issues	Identifying resources	New job/considering job change (patient, parents spouse)	Friends
Family planning issues		New relationships	Potential partners
		Adolescence	Partners
		Planning family (parents, person with bleeding dis-order, spouse)	Spouses and extended family siblings

Table 11.2 Educational Intervention Timeline

	Birth–1 year	Years 2–4	Years 5–9	Years 10–12	Years 13–18	Young Adult	Adult
Diagnosis	Review s/s bleeding treatment option	Review basics of hemophilia with child	Review: Assessment & management of bleeding episodes	Dating/Relationships	Review with pt: Genetics Prevention/safety Current management	Family planning issues Financial insurance	Review: Assessment/management Changing trends Product choice
Severity	Prevention & safety	(How blood clots and treatment works, when to tell he's hurt)	I.V. skills with parents	Genetics	Product choice Viral complications Disclosure Transmission		Employment issues Self-infusion Infection control practices
Pathophysiology	Home therapy introduction	School issues	School/sports issues	Prevention & safety	Educational/Employment issues		Genetics Complications
Genetics	Management Replacement therapy	Continue with home therapy training or review	Product choice	Partner/friend	Partner/spouse/significant other		Education of children of adult patients

(continued)

183

Table 11.2 *(continued)*

	Birth–1 year	Years 2–4	Years 5–9	Years 10–12	Years 13–18	Young Adult	Adult
Sites of Bleeding							
S/S Bleeding	Prophylaxis options	Including infection control practices	Begin self-infusion for child	Education/career planning	Pathophysiology Assessment/management of bleeding		Description of hemophilia
Treatment Options	Orthopedic complications	Financial issues	Complications of bleeding	Product choice	Infusion skills (if appropriate)		Genetics
Delivery of Care Options	Infection control practices	Product choice	Complications of treatment	Diagnostic tests; pathophysiology of hemophilia	Genetics		Future directions
Prevention & Safety	Product choice Financial issues	New therapeutic options	Social issues	Recertify home therapy skills	Complications & viral transmission		
Product Choice	Include child in simple explanation during treatment	Prevention & safety—child & parents		Prevention of viral transmission			
Diagnostic Tests	Babysitter issues			Financial issues			
Financial/Insurance							

horror stories about hemophilia, identify priorities of care, and develop a mutual plan of learning, including recognition of learning styles, interests, strengths, and barriers for each learner.

Drawing upon appropriate theoretical frameworks for educational interventions involves establishing familiarity with them and the ability to assess whether they are appropriate for a particular situation. The Health Belief Model, combined with a self-efficacy component, often is applicable in these situations. More recently, health educators have been emphasizing the value of a model involving stages of readiness to learn. Although, one should begin with the theoretical framework, real-world situations often necessitate creatively combining what should be done with what can be done in terms of available resources, time, and funding.

Introduction to Table 11.1
Core Curriculum: A Guideline to Hemophilia Education

Hemophilia education is necessary to assure optimal health for all individuals with bleeding disorders. The need for education is not limited to patients and family members; it extends to friends, caretakers, schools, employers, other community agencies, and medical providers of all disciplines. Community-based physicians, nurses, dentists, physical therapists, pharmacists, and social workers are among the health care providers for whom current education is vital.

Who does the teaching? Traditionally, we think of doctors and nurses teaching patients and families. Certainly, in the hemophilia community, that is a crucial component of learning to care for a person with a bleeding disorder; doctors and nurses at the Hemophilia Treatment Centers conduct comprehensive, ongoing patient and family education. PCPs play an important role in reinforcing education, especially for new patients. However, that is only the beginning of the process. Patients and family members become well-informed about hemophilia and have valuable experiences and insights into the disorders, their diagnosis and management.

Potential teachers include parents of children with hemophilia. Parents teach their children; they also teach other parents, physicians, and other medical providers. They teach the babysitters, the neighbors, and school staff about hemophilia. Children with hemophilia are also teachers. They share their knowledge and experience with other children with hemophilia, with their classmates, and with caregivers. Adult patients have the responsibility of educating many people about their disorder; they teach friends, partners, spouses, children, doctors, nurses, dentists, employers, and insurance carriers. In many cases, they serve as peer educators for other adults or children with hemophilia.

Hemophilia education, then, is provided by all members of the hemophilia community to each other and to the general community. The goal for each of these teachers and learners is to enhance understanding of bleeding disorders to promote optimal health for affected individuals.

A Simulated Prospective Care Study: A Continuum of Patient Education

Matthew is a 6-month-old, recently diagnosed with severe factor VIII deficiency. His parents will meet with the hemophilia nurse coordinator and identify other potential learners, such as grandparents, older siblings, or babysitters. The education will focus on the diagnosis, genetics, pathophysiology, and treatment of hemophilia. In addition, parents will receive anticipatory guidance to help them and their child adjust to living with hemophilia. Parents will be given hints to help the child develop a good self image and a sense of self-efficacy, as they are key to his success in adapting well to a chronic illness. Information will be prioritized and basics will be covered first. Emphasis will be placed on provision of a safe environment and early recognition and intervention of potential bleeding episodes.

As Matthew grows, education will continue at every encounter with the family's providers, and they will share their knowledge with pediatricians and other persons caring for the baby. Communication between community-based providers and HTC will be established and maintained throughout his life.

At some point, Matthew's parents or maternal aunts and cousins may wish to have additional information about patterns of inheritance, carrier testing, and/or prenatal diagnosis. This is provided without cost, usually during flexible hours, by the HTC nursing staff.

Education about factor replacement products, methods of delivery of products, and potential treatment protocols—such as primary prophylaxis, which often requires placement of a venous access device—will be important as Matthew approaches his first birthday.

Home therapy education will start early in life, with the suggestion of the possibility of such a program when he is a baby. Depending on his treatment requirements, the actual training for home infusions may begin when he is about 4. (Sooner if he is on primary prophylaxis; different education and timing if a central line is placed.) Both parents and, some-times, an additional caregiver are encouraged to participate in this training.

As Matthew approaches preschool age or enters a day care program, staff at the site will need education. The parents will be the primary teachers, but often will require support for additional education from the HTC staff. The emphasis here would be on child safety, activities and when and whom to notify in the event of a problem or question. Also, Matthew will need age-appropriate explanations about his treatments or other interventions.

As a school-aged child, Matthew will require ongoing education, at age level, about hemophilia; what it is, how he got it, how to stay safe, what to report to parents or teachers and what the treatment is (how does it work?). Matthew will be the one teaching his friends and teachers, by words and example, what it means to live with hemophilia.

School nurses, teachers, and physical education teachers require signifi-cant education about hemophilia. They will need to know what to expect, about any activity restrictions, method of treatment, what is an emergency, and how much time they can expect him to miss. Matthew's parents will again be the primary teachers, but a visit to the school by a medical provider will go a long way to promoting understanding and communication.

As Matthew nears 11 or 12, he may be ready to take on more responsibil-ity for his care. He already has been holding Band-Aids and rolling the factor vials; now he may wish to learn self-infusion. His parents will be the primary teachers. He will observe their technique and watch how they assess a bleed and calculate the correct dose. He may begin his participation in the process slowly, one step at a time. When he is ready, he will need formal training about assessment and treatment from the HTC staff and he will be taught proper venipuncture skills and infection control practices by the nurse at the center or by the home care nurse. Certification will be needed before he is able to complete the procedure on his own. He will be reminded how to keep accurate records about his bleeding and treatment.

About this time, Matthew may be telling his friends, coaches, or teachers about hemophilia; conducting some community education of his own.

Matthew may have girlfriends that he wishes to tell about hemophilia; serious relationships or potential sexual partners will need to have information about potential sexually transmitted viruses. Matthew may provide this information himself, with or without the help of medical providers, or he may ask his friend/partner to come to the HTC for counseling and education. Significant others may wish to help with the infusions or assessment of bleeding episodes. Health care providers will be able to help Matthew with this education, if he wishes.

Vocational/educational counseling will be important to help Matthew choose a career path that will be appropriate for him, considering his strengths, talents, preferences, and any possible limitations he has. Health care providers can be a valuable resource to help educate school staff and counselors about hemophilia, dispelling myths and advocating for Matthew. During this time, it may be necessary to teach case managers or other insurance carrier staff about hemophilia and its requirements for optimal health.

Matthew will be learning, as he grows up, about preparation for independent living; promoting wellness, safety, warning signs of bleeding, assessment and early intervention for episodes and maintaining responsibility for his health and treatment. He may need to transfer to an adult Hemophilia Treatment Center and will need guidance during this transition.

As he enters a serious relationship, Matthew's significant other may wish to participate in more formal education about hemophilia and its treatment. Issues about family planning may be important to review, as will information about safer sex and sexual transmission of potential viruses. Infection control practices should be reviewed with all household contacts. His sisters should be counseled about their potential carrier status and options available for testing.

Matthew's children will require education about hemophilia; his daughters will need to understand that they are obligate carriers. All information to children should be presented in a developmentally appropriate way. Much of this will be done by Matthew and his wife; they will guide and teach them about hemophilia as they guide them through the other paths of life as they grow up.

Conclusion

Patients and families face many challenges in coping with coagulation disorders. Health care professionals also must confront situations that are both unfamiliar and complex. Physicians who have not experienced working in a family partnership milieu, or in a multidisciplinary team setting, may have been involved only in a one-on-one doctor-patient relationship. They also may be completely unfamiliar with the concept of a community of patients and families. Potential problems that may arise for both groups are discussed in Table 11.3.

Risk Assessment

Many adult hemophilia patients and family members are highly sophisticated consumers with a broad knowledge base and strong demands. Health care professionals will benefit from the realization that families functioning as peer educators provide a cost-effective solution to a large part of the care giving situation.

Prevention of significant complications and fatalities from hemophilia relies on thorough and complete education of patients and family members. Early recognition of bleeding is the cornerstone of treatment to prevent such complications as joint disease which has been a hallmark of hemophilia. As the treatment of hemophilia has become more advanced, it has grown increasingly complicated. Patients and families are now called upon to make decisions regarding choice of treatment products and methods of care delivery. These decisions require informed consent, which only is possible when the patient and family have worked in partnership with the care providers to become well educated about all aspects of management of hemophilia or vWd.

Gaining an understanding of problems that can arise as a result of viral contamination of human plasma products is a key component of necessary knowledge. Viruses associated with blood products include hepatitis viruses: HAV, HBV, HCV, and HDV. Parvovirus and the possibility of the etiological agent of Creutzfeld-Jakob disease also may present problems.

At present, HIV and HCV are complications leading to morbidity and mortality. In addition to basic hemophilia education and therapy, these require extensive education and management. Accessing expertise from other specialties may be necessary if providers have not added these experts to the inhouse team.

All lifelong chronic conditions require continuous management. In addition to offering treatment, providers have the opportunity to enhance their health care delivery by incorporating patient and family education

Table 11.3 Risk Assessment

Type	Time Period	Patient/Family	Providers
Delay in recognition and diagnosis	Early life	No family history No preparation Possible charges of child abuse due to excessive visible bruising	Lack of awareness and expertise
Delay/difficulty in finding medical expertise	Anytime	Delayed treatment	Uncertainty
Financial costs of care	From infancy throughout life	Severe financial hardship/bankruptcy Possible forced dependency on government programs Reduced access to comprehensive care treatment centers	Defer/cancel certain types of treatment (immune tolerance, orthopedic) Over- or underutilization of factor replacement
Hemophilia (bleeding related)	Infancy on	Pain management Disruption of life	Uncertainty/lack of skill leading to over- or undertreatment Unpredictable patient demands
Complications of treatment			
Viral-hepatitis, HIV	Present in previously infected patients	Adds burden of additional chronic (sometimes fatal) chronic illness	Difficulties—skills needed in managing 2 or more chronic illnesses Potential burnout from complexity of situation Specialist referrals often indicated

(continued)

Table 11.3 (continued)

Type	Time Period	Patient/Family	Providers
Special HIV-related risks	From infection on	Transmission to sexual partner Difficulty in finding medical expertise to manage 2 chronic illnesses HIV stigma leading to social isolation	New skills/knowledge needed More provider involvement Fear of infection
Women/girls who bleed	On initial medical contact Postsurgical Postdental Menarche	Pain, life disruption Ill health	Lack of awareness of female Factor VIII and Factor IX carriers who bleed due to low levels of clotting factor and of von Willebrand's disease Need for sophisticated tests to diagnose von Willebrand's disease (lack of adherence)
Lack of understanding ("team" multidisciplinary collaborative model)		Distrust of provider's skill Feelings of exclusion Anger/hostility toward provider Denial of disease "Crisis" care only	Noncompliance from patient Poor follow-up Recurrent medical "crises"
Emergency room care	Anytime	Uniformed emergency room personnel Lack of therapeutic products Lengthy waiting time, delay in treatment Personnel do not listen to patient and family Level of pain not evaluated correctly	Lack of familiarity of bleeding problems Lack of expertise Unresponsive to expressed family expertise

into the care plan. Relevant information and the process of education are the keys to maintenance of appropriate health related behavior. Creating and maintaining a provider–patient/family partnership will facilitate the provision of education as an integral component of care.

Today with adequate treatment and an understanding of how to manage their condition, persons with hemophilia and von Willebrand disease can be well and fully functioning members of their families and communities most of the time, rarely requiring hospitalization. Children can attend school on a regular basis and adults should have infrequent absences from work. Whether they are newborns at the beginning of the maturity continuum, or HIV positive mature adults, participation in an educational partnership will maximize their potential for a better quality of life. Provider participants also will benefit from a more satisfying practice, knowing that they have enabled their patients to be higher functioning, and to reach their health care goals. Participation in an educational partnership will maximize opportunities for achieving high quality care while maintaining a cost-effective approach.

Chapter 12

A Managed Care Model for End-of-Life Care

Daniel R. Tobin and James E. Conlon, Jr.

There is a great opportunity to incorporate comprehensive end-of-life programs into managed care settings, and some of the most innovative and effective end-of-life programs can be found in managed care organizations.

Excellent reviews of the potential benefits as well as the dangers of end-of-life programs in managed care are presented by Rousseau (1998) and Miles, Weber, and Koepp (1995). The current opportunity to implement innovative and far-reaching programs for individuals with advanced illness within managed care far outweigh the potential conflicts. However, due to the cost containment strategies of managed care companies, public leaders as well as many practitioners have concern about access to resources and information in managed care, especially at the end of life (Kuczewski, 1998).

An abundance of evidence demonstrates the need to improve care at the end of life within the American health care system. The publication of the Support Study in 1995 (The Support Principal Investigators, 1995) followed by the Institute of Medicine's "Approaching Death: Improving Care at the End of Life" demonstrated that the current medical system too often lacks the training and perspective to offer patients a peaceful, comfortable end of life, and that "too many people suffer from pain and other distress that clinicians could prevent or relieve" (Field & Cassel, 1997).

To help patients transition from advancing illness into the dying process, end-of-life treatments and programs need to integrate comprehensive, interdisciplinary efforts into mainstream medical practice. Rather than being restricted to the last weeks or months of life, effective programs must take a wide view of the dying process and help individuals, their families, and loved ones find tranquility in facing serious illness. The hospice movement and palliative care medicine have done an excellent job of pioneering good end-of-life care. However, despite the growth of the hospice movement, only 17% of Americans die with hospice care and, in most parts of the country, the length of stay is very short (Financing Task Force Retreat, 1998). What we need now is to take what the hospice movement has done and expand it so that people can die in hospitals, homes, and hospices with the same level of comfort and care.

Currently, many new programs which focus on developing standards for good end-of-life care are being instituted and evaluated. Dying well can be defined as maintaining dignity, control, pain management, and continued development of one's psychosocial, and spiritual self to the very end.

Innovative programs are being supported by the Robert Wood Johnson Foundation, The Project on Death In America, The National V.A. Health Care System, The Nathan Cummings Foundation, and The Center to Improve Care of the Dying at George Washington University, as well as many community groups and national educational efforts. At the core of all of these programs is the fact that dying well can be defined and measured by specific criteria, and the assumption that, if given the chance, it is something most of us would want for ourselves and those we love.

There is a need for consumer involvement in the development and expansion of national end-of-life programs. The American public must begin to focus on demanding proper pain management as well as information and guidance with end-of-life issues. The Partnership for Caring, a national consumer group, is spearheading legislative and consumer education efforts in these areas. The "Advance Planning and Compassionate Care Act of 1997," introduced by Senator Rockefeller and Senator Collins, is an excellent attempt for government leaders to require health care facilities to provide information in advanced illness planning.

End-of-life programs, as well as all health care delivery, need to be seen as a public policy issue rather than primarily a financial agenda. Managed care inherently requires a focus on managing costs, but health care choices must be made with the realization that the nature of our national health care delivery system defines the nature of our public policy.

Our culture's emerging recognition of peaceful dying will create a demand for and openness to programs that help people die with dignity and comfort. A culture that routinely uses methods of peaceful dying will in time see that such programs have a strong effect on the entire community.

Managed care organizations need to create end-of-life programs that are comprehensive, community-based, and integrated within their entire delivery system. Comprehensive programs must incorporate a broad view of the dying process, involving the patient, family and loved ones, physicians, nurses, social workers, and other health care providers as well as the entire community. In developing community input to end-of-life programs, it is helpful to include community focus groups such as those reported in The American Health Decision's publication entitled "The Quest To Die with Dignity" and the Allina Foundation's "Project Decide." It is imperative to involve local religious and spiritual groups, as well as the needs of diverse cultural groups and pediatric populations.

End-of-life programs need to incorporate the availability of all aspects of medical and surgical care, pain management, and symptom control, as well as psychosocial and spiritual needs. Dr. Ira Bycock, a hospice pioneer and consumer advocate, has demonstrated the importance of improving and measuring end of life care while understanding "The Nature of Suffering and the Nature of Opportunity at the End of Life" (Bycock, 1996). In forming comprehensive community-based end-of-life programs it would be wise to incorporate and research the biopsychosocial model proposed by Engel (1977).

All new programs must be developed with operational detail that allows them to be portable to other communities. A successful program in one location does not assure that it can automatically work in another community unless it is planned with that goal. It is intuitive that well-structured end-of-life programs will improve end-of-life care and yield significant secondary savings. However, carefully planned, controlled research will define and demonstrate specific outcomes.

We present a model comprehensive, community-based end-of-life program which is in operation and being studied in several locations throughout the country. The FairCare Health System (FCHS) as it is called, is an operational model based on the FairCare Program (Tobin, 1999) which is outlined in the book entitled "Peaceful Dying: The Step-By-Step Guide to Preserving Your Dignity, Your Choice and Your Inner Peace at the

End of Life." This program creates a standard psychosocial model for end-of-life care and moves the clinical intervention to the time of diagnosis with an end of life situation. The FairCare program integrates with mainstream medical care and is structured to be collaborative with other end-of-life care models.

The program relies on a collaborative care model which trains and supervises a single nurse practitioner to use the FairCare program within managed care. The nurse practitioner is backed by a social worker and medical director who are trained in the standardized communication model. Each team consisting of nurse practitioner, social worker, and medical director can see approximately 200 patients a year.

The FairCare program is based on the premise that a standard communication model for conversations at the end of life is essential in order to overcome our cultural difficulties with facing the subject of dying. The program offers a flexible A-Z, step-by-step guide for events and decisions at the end of life which include the importance of maintaining individuality and dignity, confronting fear of dying, pain management, and family as well as physician support. FairCare discourages suicide and notes that most people are searching for comprehensive health care which addresses the physical, psychological, and spiritual aspects of dying. The program posits that dying is a natural part of living and focuses on helping individual patients maintain control of their decisions and find "the Turning Point" or "Window of Opportunity" where an advanced illness becomes the dying process and comfort care may be requested.

Initially piloted and studied with the VA Health Care Network Upstate NY, FCHS utilizes the FairCare program to operationalize a comprehensive, clinical, community-based end of life program. The system currently is in operation in managed care organizations, nursing homes, and community groups throughout the country. Initially, care managers within an organization are identified and trained in the FairCare program so that they can provide information and guidance to patients and family members facing advancing illness. The FairCare program's standard communication model then is introduced through a public education campaign. In order to familiarize all clinicians with the program, medical, nursing, and healthcare worker education is provided to the managed care organization staff.

The patient education and empowerment campaign utilizes patient education brochures, community study groups, and community meetings to introduce the FairCare concepts. These efforts are not meant to glamorize a

Hollywood illusion of peaceful dying, but rather to familiarize community members with the terrain of terminal illness. Public education and empowerment helps the public take responsibility for having realistic expectations, and provides the tools necessary for facing end-of-life care within managed care settings.

FairCare education and training utilizes marker based presentations in order to categorize the FairCare Program into 5 basic phases (Table 12.1). The first phase is "Individuality of Disease" followed by phase 2, "Confronting Fear." The third phase is labeled "Practical Issues," which include steps C through K. The fourth and pivotal phase is "The Turning Point," which includes being ready to acknowledge that an advanced illness has become the dying process and that continued curative efforts probably will not be helpful to most people. This allows an individual, in partnership with his or her family, loved ones, and physicians, to shift to the fifth phase, "Finding Peace," which includes steps N-Z of the FairCare program.

The FairCare model is structured as an adjunct service, which requires minimal additional resources for financing and allows patients to remain with all of their health care providers. The care manager's role, with physician and social work support, is to be focused on an empowered, individualized patient's decision being integrated into the care plan on a daily basis. The FairCare program also is available in physician and staff education brochures for all clinicians within a managed care setting.

Due to the comprehensive and flexible nature of this model program, we are gathering outcome data on the integration of the FCHS within managed care settings, and demonstrating increased utilization of palliative care; patient, family, and caregiver satisfaction; improved pain and symptom control; secondary cost savings, and improved access to and quality of end-of-life care. Preliminary data demonstrate a trend toward reduction in fear of death among a pilot group of patients. The public's demand for improved end-of-life care, as well as the health care system's responsibility to create new palliative care programs, support our recommendations that managed care parties that bear the financial risk for health care services create an insurance reimbursement model for these services.

The insurance reimbursement model must recognize that the fundamental goal of FCHS is to fulfill the public's demand for improved end-of-life care. By definition, this goal must focus the delivery of care on improving the quality of life to terminally ill patients and their loved ones. The financing and delivery of such a program should be provided

Table 12.1   A Standardized Communication Model for End-of-Life Care

Phase 1: Individuality of Disease
   A.   Recognizing Individuality of Disease, Individuality of Choice

Phase 2: Confronting Fear
   B.   Confronting, Expressing and Diminishing Fear of Dying

Phase 3: Practical Issues
   C.   Slowing Down Time and the Mind
   D.   Creating Positive Days
   E.   Talking to Your Doctor—the Early Stages
   F.   Talking to Your Family
   G.   Coming to Terms with this Reality
   H.   Seeking Counseling and Support
   I.   Selecting Advance Directives
   J.   Considering Other Practical Concerns
   K.   Examining Spiritual View on Living and Dying

Phase 4: the Turning Point
   L.   Being Ready
   M.   Shifting to Care

Phase 5: Finding Peace
   N.   Ensuring Family Support
   O.   Talking to Your Doctor Again
   P.   Dealing with the Suicide Questions
   Q.   Deciding Where to Die
   R.   Getting Relief for Your Pain
   S.   Dealing with Physical Changes
   T.   Nurturing Your Body, Mind, and Spirit
   U.   Telling Your Story
   V.   Embracing Love as the Meaning of Life
   W.   Achieving Peace of Mind
   X.   Helping Plan Your Funeral or Memorial Service
   Y.   Preparing Your Loved Ones for Their Bereavement
   Z.   Dying with Tranquility

through a case management model, with the caregiver functioning solely as an advocate for the terminally ill patient's overall well-being in end-of-life decision making. In this capacity the caregiver's goals are aligned with those of the patient, the family, the provider, and ultimately, those of the plan sponsor and third-party payer.

The case management model, which is focused on outcome, avoids the contentious managed care policy issue of rationing or denying care in the interest of maximizing profits. Case management provides the best opportunity to realize the FCHS goals for the patient while at the same time achieving substantial savings for the plan sponsor and third party payer, by focusing the scarce resources of the integrated medical delivery system to the most clinically appropriate cases.

Reimbursement of the case manager on a salaried or a time-charge basis removes the caregiver from the issue of maximizing the savings to the financially at-risk parties. Successful implementation of FCHS through case management insurance reimbursement will improve end-of-life care, as well as create actuarial efficiencies by refocusing and redirecting intensive and costly medical resources in the financing of health care and employee benefits. Improved access to care resulting from more affordable public and private health insurance is a likely byproduct of successfully implementing the FCHS through the case management insurance reimbursement model.

In summary, there is a great opportunity to implement innovative end-of-life programs within managed care. These programs need to be comprehensive, community-based, and integrated within the spectrum of services provided by health systems. The FairCare Health system and FairCare program are presented as a clinical model for putting a standard communication model for end-of-life care into operation. Several methods of insurance reimbursement are proposed. The current challenge is for all managed care organizations to implement, evaluate, and refine programs which improve end-of-life care for their members. As Engel (1977) noted in his seminal work, "In a free society, outcome will depend upon those who have the courage to try new paths and the wisdom to provide the necessary support" (p. 196).

PART III
Looking Ahead

Chapter 13

We Need Partners: Forging Strong Relationships with Patients

S. Jody Heymann and Christine Kerr

Troubled Relationships: Inadequate Information-Sharing, Problem Solving, and Decision Making

Dr. Schultz told Sara, "Sam will need to take antibiotics daily to prevent further infections, at least until he can have a test to see if there is reflux," referring to the backward flow of urine from the bladder to the kidneys. "If he does have reflux, he'll need to take daily antibiotics for at least a year." Sarah wanted to know the reasoning behind the physician's recommendations so she could decide what was best for her newborn son. She asked a number of questions in order to understand: "What does the test involve? . . . What happens if Sam does not take antibiotics? . . . Do daily antibiotics in a young infant affect the development of the immune system?" But Dr. Schultz would neither answer Sarah's questions directly nor respond honestly that he did not know the answers to some of the questions, that

Portions of this chapter have appeared in print before and were excerpted with permission from the following articles:

Heymann SJ. "Patients in Research: Not Just Subjects, but Partners." *Science.* 269 (5225):797–8, 1995. Aug 11. Copyright 1995 American Association for the Advancement of Science.

Heymann SJ. "Building Partnerships with Patients." *Annals of Allergy, Asthma, and Immunology.* 78 (1-4) January 1997. Copyright 1997 Annals of Allergy, Asthma, and Immunology.

Heymann SJ. "Providing Patients with the Information They Need." Joint Commission Journal on Quality Improvement. 23(8):443-8, 1997 Aug. Copyright Joint Commission Journal on Quality Improvement. Oakbrook Terrace, IL: Joint Commission on Accreditation of Healthcare Organizations, 1997, 5.

he was not sure anyone knew the answers to those questions. Instead, he tried to frighten Sarah into following his recommendations. Sarah tried again to get information: "How common is reflux in boys that have had just one urinary tract infection?" Her questions reflected her training in research. Dr. Schultz did not answer. He walked away, asking sarcastically, "Is Sam going to grow up to be an epidemiologist?" He was indignant about being pressed for information. (Heymann, 1995)

The signs are clear—in both inpatient and outpatient settings. While many patient-provider relationships are successful and fruitful, too many are failing for us to ignore the problem. In a national survey of hospitalized patients, 32% reported that they did not know whom to ask for help if they needed it. Thirty percent said they were not told about important side effects of medicines. Twenty-eight percent reported that nurses were overworked and too busy to care for patients. Thirty-nine percent felt they did not have a relationship of trust with any hospital staff other than the doctor in charge of their care. The communication problems also affected patients after they left the hospital. Twenty-seven percent of patients reported that they were not told what danger signals to watch for at home. Twenty-four percent were not told when they could resume normal activities following hospitalization (Cleary et al., 1991).

Other research has echoed these findings and demonstrated that doctors markedly overestimate how much their patients understand when discharged. Doctors in one study thought that 89% of their just-discharged patients understood the side effects of the medicines they were taking and that 95% of the patients knew when to resume normal activities. Only 57% of their patients said that they actually knew the side effects of their medicines, and 58% knew when they could resume normal activities (Calkins, Davis, & Reiley, 1997).

Research on the experience of patients and their families outside of hospitals is equally striking. Over half of the parents of outpatients who were surveyed in one study stated that they needed to know more about both their child's diagnosis and treatment. As striking as the number of parents who felt they had inadequate information was the disparity between parents' perceptions and the perceptions of the doctors who cared for their children. When the doctors were surveyed, fewer than 1 in 12 stated that the parents needed to know more about their children's diagnosis. Less than 1 in 30 stated that the parents needed to know more about their children's treatment (Lipstak & Revell, 1989).

While changes in current health care financing have dramatically stressed doctor-patient relationships, problems in communication are not new. A study conducted almost 25 years ago found that 45% of mothers who brought their sick children to a pediatrician left not knowing what treatment their child should receive, and 30% left not knowing when their child should return to the doctor (Decastro, 1972).

Communication gaps may result in part from the different understanding patients and doctors have of the relative importance of communication in the doctor-patient relationship. In one recent study, when both patients and doctors were asked to rank the relative importance of several aspects of care, researchers found that doctors rated the provision of information the sixth most important element of care, in contrast to patients, who ranked it the second most important element—only after clinical skill (Laine, Davidoff, & Lewis, 1996).

Although one popular medical myth argues that patients don't want to know about their conditions and their treatment, data contradicting this have been available for a number of years (Nease & Brooks, 1995). Research has shown that 99% of patients want to know "what the treatment will accomplish," 98% of patients want to know the side effects of their treatments, and over 95% want to know "exactly what the treatment will do" inside their bodies (Cassileth, Zupdis, Sutton-Smith, & March, 1980).

The majority of patients feel that deciding what is done about their medical condition should be a shared decision between both the doctor and the patient (Deber, Kraetschmer, & Irvine, 1996; Mazur & Hickam, 1997). Despite this evidence, in practice, many more patients feel they have too little control over their treatment than feel they have too much control (Degner, Krisjanson, & Bowman, 1997).

Patients care enough that they change physicians when their physicians do not communicate well, or when they spend too little time with patients because of volume requirements (Kasteler, Kane, & Olsen, 1976; Marquis et al., 1983). Whether patients are involved in decision making also affects whether they change physicians. One study ranked physicians by their participatory decision-making style and showed that of the patients of doctors who were most likely to involve them in decisions, only 15% changed doctors in a year. By contrast, about one-third of the patients of the physicians who had the least participatory decision-making style changed doctors within a year (Kaplan, Greenfield, Gandek, Rogers, & Ware, 1996). There is a substantial body of evidence showing that patients fare better when they are informed about their health condition and involved in decisions about their care. The time doctors spend with patients and their willingness to involve patients in decisions has been shown to significantly affect patients' decisions about their care (Bradbury, Kay, Tighe, & Hewison, 1994; Silliman, Troyan, Guadagnoli, & Kaplan, 1997). Informing patients and encouraging patient participation has been shown to lead to decreased need for medication, decreased discomfort, shorter recovery times, and shorter lengths of hospital stay, as well as a more rapid return to work (Brody et al., 1989; Finkler & Correa, 1996; Kaplan, Greenfield, & Ware, 1989; Lerman et al., 1990; Lewis, Pantell, & Sharp, 1991).

Perhaps the single most troubling sign of problems in patient-provider relationships is the frequency with which medical treatment plans are not followed. Approximately half of all patients do not take medication as recommended (Jones, 1983). Lifestyle changes, even when explicitly recommended by a physician, are even less likely to be followed (Butler, Rollnick, & Stott, 1996; Kravitz et al., 1993). Whether or not patients follow physician recommendations has been shown to be tied to whether or not physicians demonstrate that they respect their patients, understand their patients' concerns, inform patients about both their illness and their treatment, and involve patients in developing a plan of treatment (Gondolf, 1987; Stoeckle, 1993).

While patients of any race, class, gender, or health status can and do experience communication problems in our health care system, there is little doubt that some patients are at far greater risk. National surveys of patients have found that problems are most frequent between doctors and low-income patients, patients belonging to a minority, women, and those patients in greatest need of quality relationships—patients in the poorest health (Brody, 1980; Cleary et al., 1991a; Rohling & Binder, 1995; Street, 1992).

Finding Solutions

Achievable changes in clinical practice, education, research, and evaluation of services can help address these problems.

Medical Practice

In a talk to physicians who had been practicing medicine for 25 years, Dr. Lesley Heafitz, who had been diagnosed with cancer, spoke about being a patient. She opened her comments by saying, "Someday, every single one of you, sooner or later, will become a patient. And, I daresay, you will not particularly like being on the other side of the fence" (Symposium on the Patient-Provider Relationship, 1992).

Even when health care providers are aware of the importance of informing patients about their conditions and incorporating patients' perspectives in decisions about their own care, it can be difficult to do. Several simple steps can make a big difference.

Recognizing Patient Expertise

> Vivian described telling her obstetrician that she thought her baby was about to be born, that she could feel the head coming down her vagina. He did not believe her and so did not do a physical exam. Minutes later, he and the delivery nurses were unprepared when the baby was born "precipitously." It was only precipitous to them because the obstetrician had not listened to Vivian. (Heymann, 1995)

The first step is to recognize that while physicians know more about anatomy, pathophysiology, pharmacology, and all medical sciences than do the majority of their patients, patients bring a critical complementary expertise. Patients know more than their providers about their daily lives, values, goals and priorities, as well as about their symptoms and side effects of treatment. The information that patients bring to the process is critical to making a good clinical decision. If most health conditions had a single treatment that was 100% effective and caused no side effects, then patients' values would become far less important. Patients could come into the office with their complaint, and physicians could provide a magic pill to solve it. Unfortunately, that is far from our present state. As almost all treatments have side effects and varying chances of failure, the "right" prescription depends on the patient's goals, and the impact of the disease and the treatment side effects on the patient's life. The same side effect of a medication—inability to drive is just one example—could affect the life of one patient markedly if she needed to drive to work, and yet have little effect on another patient who walked most places he needed to go.

Building Partnerships

> John had received treatment for infertility. He described a meeting he attended of fertility specialists at which doctors proposed putting three eggs in a dish with an

anonymous donor's sperm and three with a husband's sperm. The "problem" for the doctors was that some couples wanted to give the husband's sperm a better chance of fertilizing the egg by exposing four eggs to the husband's sperm and only two eggs to the donor's sperm. The doctors' goal was to get the woman pregnant regardless of who was the biologic father. The couples' goal was to conceive a child that had both the husband and wife as biologic parents. Why, he wondered, couldn't the doctors understand the parents' point of view? (Heymann, 1995, p. 6)

The second step is building a partnership with your patients (Heymann, 1995). The process of working together with the patient and making decisions is as important as the information gathered. No questionnaire filled out by the patient in the waiting room will substitute for working together. The data are clear. As discussed above, health improves significantly more rapidly in patients who participate actively in decisions about their own care. While the research is there to substantiate this, it only takes putting oneself in the patient's shoes to imagine what a difference it makes. Partnerships will require learning from, not just about, patients. It is particularly important to learn from patients about what happens to them after they leave the office or the hospital. The time that medicine most frequently fails patients is when they are discharged from the hospital or sent home from the office and the treatment that made sense at the bedside or in the examining room is impractical or impossible in their daily life (Cleary et al., 1991).

Providers need to be involved in learning from patients, teaching patients, and involving patients in their own care, but they don't need to be the only ones involved. While there are numerous examples of programs that promote patient education and participation, it is worth describing the data on a few examples. These examples share three features: actively educating patients about their health condition, providing ongoing opportunities for patients to continue to learn, and helping to provide patients with specific ways they can become more actively involved in their own care.

Examples of Specific Approaches

Effective and simple one-on-one approaches have been developed to increase patients' understanding of their health conditions and participation in their own care. In "Coached Care," Kaplan and colleagues (1989) trained lay individuals to sit down with patients, show the patients their medical charts, discuss with them ways decisions were made about managing their disease, and help the patients prepare to raise questions and concerns with their physicians. The coaching sessions lasted only 20 minutes, and did not have to be done by health professionals; these two facts contributed to their low cost. In a randomized controlled experiment, those patients who were shown their own charts and encouraged to participate actively in their own care were found to have significantly more rapid improvement in health than those who received routine care.

Effective approaches also have been used with groups of patients. Lorig and colleagues (1996) have worked with patients with a variety of chronic health conditions, including arthritis, stroke, heart and lung disease in a 14-hour Chronic Disease Self-Management Program. In this program, trained lay leaders meet in seven 2-hour sessions with patients to help them develop the skills needed to become actively involved in managing their health problems. In a randomized controlled study, patients who participated in the Disease Self-Management Program were found to spend significantly fewer days in the hospital, have significantly greater improvement in their functioning and in their communication with health care providers (Lorig, 1996).

Good and bad technological innovations in patient education abound. The best innovations provide for ongoing patient education (not just one-time opportunities) and facilitate active involvement by patients in decisions about their own care. The Comprehensive Health Enhancement Support System (CHESS), a computer system provided to patients, is one such innovation. The computer is made available to patients in their homes for a period of several months during which time they can access the information and other individuals on this system as frequently as they choose. CHESS has been tested with patients with less than a high-school education. As the computer is provided, no home computer is necessary. Patients do not need any prior computer experience.

The computer system offers a wide range of options available through a simple point-and-click procedure. Patients can choose to learn more about their disease through basic descriptions or read detailed articles about their condition in a reference library. For highly specialized questions, they can write questions to experts who will respond to them rapidly. Patients can use decision aids to assist them in making choices for their own care. They can read about the experiences of other patients with their disease, and they can choose whether or not to participate in a computer discussion group with others who have the same disease. Gustafson and colleagues demonstrated that having the use of CHESS significantly improved the quality of life of patients, not only in the period when the computer was in their home and they had access to it, but afterward. Hospital costs per patient who was living with an HIV infection declined more than $200 per month in a controlled experiment. Hospital costs remained lower for patients even when they no longer had the computer (Gustafson et al., 1994). The presumed mechanism for this was the patients' higher level of knowledge about their disease and involvement in their own care subsequent to their having access to CHESS. HIV-infected people of different backgrounds, ages, genders, ethnicities, and disease states used the computer frequently, showing that the system was useful even to those who were especially at risk for not having a strong patient-doctor partnership (Pingree, Hawkins, & Gustafson, 1994). CHESS also has been useful for women who were diagnosed with breast cancer. A study of minority women in two different neighborhoods indicated that the subjects felt more positive emotions, such as relief, understanding, and empowerment, and fewer negative emotions, such as stress, boredom, and fear after using CHESS (McTavish et al., 1994).

Technology also can make it easier for the physician to involve the patient in his or her care. The simple change of allowing physicians to enter patient preferences into a computerized patient record so that other doctors will be aware of the preferences is one such innovation currently being investigated (Caspar & Brennan, 1994).

Patient Participation in Research

Like clinical care, medical research would be better able to help serve patients if patients were more involved in the research process as partners both at early stages, when research questions are being formulated, and at later stages, when recommendations are formulated based on research results.

In the past, patients or non-health professionals were asked to represent patient views on institutional review boards. Although these initiatives may be valuable, they have been limited in two important ways. First, patients often are asked to give a generalist's perspective. They review research about health conditions they have not experienced. Secondly, patients often have been asked to approve or disapprove the use of human research subjects or the quality of informed consent for research projects that already have been designed.

At the Earliest Stages: Determining What Issues Will Be Studied

As researchers, we could all improve the quality and relevance of our research by spending more time at the early stages of study design talking with the people we hope our research will help. Often laboratory studies, social science surveys, or clinical trials are designed with the input only of researchers. This is because we recognize the expertise that researchers have. What we have failed to adequately recognize is that patients have a complementary expertise.

Researchers know more than most patients about how to design a sound study to answer a particular question. Researchers can build on their scientific knowledge and develop proposals for treatment that many patients can not. At the same time, patients can draw on their experience of their illness and past treatments, and think of questions that researchers need to answer—questions that may not occur to the majority of researchers.

Research would change in a number of ways if we spent more time listening to patients while we were designing studies. If patients' concerns were addressed, there would be more research on the side effects of treatments. In general, physicians grossly underestimate patients "functional disabilities" or symptoms (Calkins et al., 1991). Patients' desires to know how treatments affect the quality of their lives can be better addressed in research. Reliable and valid measures of patients' experiences of mental, emotional, and social functioning have been developed (Cleary, Greenfield, & McNeil, 1991; Jette et al., 1986; Stewart, Greenfield, & Hays, 1989; Tarlov et al., 1989). These should be used in conjunction with physiological indicators to assess possible treatment choices.

If patients were involved in the early stages of research design, the outcomes studied would be different. Physicians developing in vitro fertilization have studied the question of how many patients who made it to the stage of embryo transfer went on to have positive pregnancy tests. Although answering this question is valuable and may be readily done, it will not enable researchers to answer the question people who are deciding whether or not to have in vitro fertilization often pose: if we try in vitro fertilization, what are our chances of giving birth to a baby? An embryo transplant depends on an embryo harvest, which is not possible in all cases. Not everyone who has a positive pregnancy test is able to carry the fetus to term and give birth to a live baby. To answer those patients who want to know their chances of giving birth, a study would need, at the same time, to measure the probability that people who enter in vitro fertilization programs get pregnant and give birth to a live child.

More long-term research is needed to address patient concerns. Industrialized countries are now countries of chronic diseases. Major killers of the past, including infant mortality and acute infections, now kill far fewer in the United States. The major killers of today—heart disease and cancer—are chronic diseases, as are major causes of morbidity, such as asthma and epilepsy. Not only has the decline in acute illnesses left chronic diseases as the major causes of death and disability, but the increased longevity of the population means that more people are living lengthy periods with chronic non-fatal ailments. Yet research still focuses on the short-run benefits and side effects of treatments. Research funding and institutions are not structured in a way to permit long-term research. Researchers are called upon to show results in 3 years, not 30. Patients' lives work on a different time frame. Patients with chronic conditions often know they will be living with a particular disease, its symptoms, the treatment, and its side effects for the rest of their lives. They need information about both immediate treatment choices and long term consequences. Hearing patients' concerns about what questions need to be answered could help balance the need for both short- and long-term research.

At the End of Research: How Patients' Perspectives May Affect Recommendations

Similarly, patient input at the final stages of research could significantly improve its usefulness to patients. Recommendations based on study results typically are formulated by researchers and clinicians in discussions in which patients are absent. The absence of patients in the formulation of uniform recommendations is particularly striking, given the body of research which demonstrates that the value of a treatment often depends on the patient. Using analytic methods, researchers have demonstrated that in many instances there is no one treatment that is objectively better for all patients; the best treatment depends on the patient's values and how the patient weighs the risks and benefits of the treatment (Barry, 1988). In presenting treatment recommendations without incorporating the values of patients, researchers' values are inherently used to balance the risks and benefits of any treatment. In presenting uniform recommendations as opposed to information to assist patients in making decisions, investigators often inadvertently obscure the fact that the best treatment choice depends on the individual patient's values and preferences.

Although research results generally are presented in rooms absent of the patients they affect, there are exceptions. One of these is in the field of AIDS research. Unusual cases of unfair or inhumane treatment of researchers by protesters may have obscured the wide benefits of having patients present at many AIDS conferences. The presence of people living with AIDS at meetings discussing research leaves an indelible stamp on what takes place. There is a constant reminder of how the proposed research affects the lives of individuals. Their presence affects both what subjects are proposed for study, the design of research proposals, interpretations, and policy recommendations made based on the results.

In contrast, much recent tuberculosis research has been done without patient input. At one meeting, investigators and policy makers presented a proposal to require every single person who is diagnosed with tuberculosis to have a professional present for each pill they take in treatment (directly observed therapy (DOT)). The rationale was that the imposition on infected individuals would be trivial and the public health gains great. Yet, the details of the program were not spelled out. DOT can mean anything from a health care worker coming to the home of the patient twice a week for 9 months, to the person with tuberculosis being required to go the doctor's office or clinic daily. DOT continues to be widely recommended as cost-effective, with little attention being paid to the costs borne by patients. Given that most patients with tuberculosis do take their medicine as instructed the burden of DOT could be quite substantial, as well as unnecessary, for a mother of three children, with no one to share their care, who lives an hour by bus from the clinic.

Patient Participation at Every Stage

The beginning and end of the research process are only two examples of times when patient participation would be valuable. There are roles that patients can play at every stage of research, and their knowledge can complement that of researchers. Clinical trials frequently need to address problems that lead to patients being unwilling to sign up for a study, or to continue in a study once they have begun. Research has shown that when patients are included in decision making from the start, they are more likely to participate in clinical trials (Ruckdeschel, Albrecht, Blanchard, & Hemmick, 1996). Carey and Smith also have reported on an innovative and valuable use of patients in focus groups and a participatory advisory panel (Carey & Smith, 1992). Patients provided information that was important to the researchers' ability both to recruit study subjects and to obtain unbiased information.

Learning from Patients

Including patients as subjects in clinical trials should be only one of the ways in which patients have a chance to participate (McNeill, 1993). Together we could better define which research questions should be studied, determine what outcomes should be measured, encourage patient participation in adherence to protocols, and interpret what research results mean for the daily lives of patients. In the process of eliciting patients' viewpoints, it is important that no one person be asked to represent all patients. Patients' experiences and viewpoints vary as much from each others' as they do from researchers'. Patients' viewpoints can be elicited on a one-time basis in focus groups and on an ongoing basis through advisory panels. Much can be learned from experiences over the past 15 years in clinical medicine. Patients have welcomed the opportunity to become more involved in their own clinical care. The quality of research would be greatly enriched and patients better served if they were welcomed as partners, not just subjects, in research.

Medical Education

> Silva had cancer. He was young and had been perfectly healthy a year before. The first physician who cared for him had failed to detect his cancer. When chemotherapy was started, it worked temporarily, but the cancer soon returned. We sat and talked shortly after his relapse. He was one of the patients doctors talk about being pained to see. Silva said simply, "The more training the doctors get, the more they stay away from me and won't talk to me." (Heymann, 1995, p. 237)

Numerous medical schools teach little or nothing in the classroom about the impact of illness on patients' daily lives, and about the importance to patients' health of being informed about their conditions and involved in decision making. The first thing that can be done in medical education is to use this research to dispel incorrect myths, and to educate medical students about the importance of patient involvement in their own care.

Talking about the importance will not be enough; educational programs need to demonstrate it. At present, most case presentations—in the classroom and in the ward—describe a patient's symptoms, detail the physical exam and laboratory values, then ask for "the best" diagnostic plan and treatment. National board exams ask for single answers out of multiple choices. Rarely do either lessons or tests describe a patient's values, his daily life, his goals, or how these might affect the best diagnostic or therapeutic plan. Little attention is paid to the process by which therapeutic decisions are made, e.g., the extent to which the patient is involved in decision making about his own care. (Ironically, the one exception to this is the case of dying patients, for whom the standard of care has become informing and involving patients and their families in decisions not to resuscitate.) Patients themselves are rarely seen in preclinical years, and when they are seen in clinical years they are seen as a source of information about symptoms, as bodies to examine for physical exam signs, and as bodies on which to conduct diagnostic tests. In grand rounds, patients are frequently invited to describe their symptoms and then asked to leave while those present discuss possible diagnostic and treatment plans.

Ward teaching consists of rounding "on" patients—an apt preposition. The attending, medical students and residents walk in; a physical finding is often demonstrated; they then leave for their discussion. But there are many ways the patients could be involved in medical education. How simple it would be, yet how radical, if even once a week rounds focused on the experience of patients in the hospital, on how their hospital treatment affected their lives outside the hospital. How different grand rounds would look if they routinely incorporated the patient's perspective on the care they received.

Many of the schools that take important steps in the classroom drop the ball when it comes to the wards. Medical students need to learn more from patients and their families on the wards, in clinics, and in the community about the experience of illness and health care directly. At the Children's Hospital of Philadelphia, parents teach physicians about the impact of illness on their children's lives. This program is only one of a number that have demonstrated the willingness of patients and families to be involved in teaching on the ward.

Training can play an important role for physicians in practice as well as for medical students. One intervention which simply provided feedback to doctors about how to improve "patient-doctor concordance"—the agreement between patients and doctors about symptoms, diagnosis, treatment, and expectations—showed that even a small intervention resulted in better communication between doctors and patients (Liaw, Young, & Farish, 1996). Another intervention showed that briefly training doctors to improve their communication skills significantly reduced patients' anxiety and emotional distress (Roter et al., 1995). A study which gave physicians 4.5 hours of training on how to involve patients in their care also showed positive results from both the doctors' and the patients' perspectives (Joos, Hickam, Gordon, & Baker, 1996).

Health Care System

> Bill had just been diagnosed with stomach cancer. He went to the hospital to have a highly specialized test, which would determine whether the cancer involved all layers of his stomach, performed. That finding would reveal how long he had to live. The oncologist who told him that the cancer had grown through the entire stomach wall spent only five minutes with him. Five minutes to tell him that he had a 10 to 20 percent chance of survival and that to get that chance he would need to have radical surgery. "Oh," the oncologist replied to Bill's request for names of good surgeons, "Anyone can do the surgery." He must have meant anyone with experience in that type of cancer surgery. Bill had no idea how to find such a surgeon. Then the oncologist was gone, and Bill was alone with his problem. (Heymann, 1995, p. 5)

Overall, nearly half of all outpatient visits provided by any physician last less than 10 minutes, and the average visit lasts just 12 minutes (Stoeckle, 1993). Not only are longer visits more humane when dealing with life-and-death issues, but when doctors spend more time with patients dealing with common illnesses, they are more likely to involve patients in decisions about their care (Kaplan et al., 1996). Doctors' appointments need to be set up to last more than an average of 12 minutes so that physicians can learn that they can afford to listen and that their patients cannot afford for them not to listen. The evidence is there. By decreasing the duration of hospitalization, patient involvement can lead to reduced inpatient costs as well as higher quality care. Costs can also be cut by involving patients in outpatient care. High blood pressure and high blood sugar are only two examples of conditions that, when poorly controlled, can lead to poor health and the need for expensive care. Both hypertension and diabetes are better controlled after brief interventions to increase the role individuals play in their medical care beyond that of a compliant patient (Greenfield, Kaplan, Ware, Yano, & Frank, 1989). When doctors spend more time with patients, they not only can provide better care, but they can save the costs of unnecessary tests and interventions, which often inadequately and expensively replace communication. They also can save the cost of avoidable misdiagnosis, mistreatment, and patient misunderstanding that lie in the wake of dispatch.

While individual physicians often have little say over how much time they spend with patients, physician groups can influence the time individual physicians have with patients. Physicians can use their own strength and the strength of their professional organizations to ensure that they can provide humane care.

The economics of health care need to be reformed. Current paradigms for cost-cutting pit patients against insurers, and often place physicians in the middle of the tug-of-war. We can improve quality without increasing costs. The solution is neither magic nor an ephemeral image produced by smoke and mirrors. It requires an investment—this time, in patients.

Quality Improvement

Academics have long used a series of quality measures of health plans including process measures, outcome measures, and measures of access. However, patients choosing plans, hospitals, and physicians have had little access to measures of quality. As a result, plans have competed primarily on the basis of cost. Recently, a wide range of national organizations have been developing quality measures that they hope will be used widely by plans and made available to consumers. These initiatives have the chance to affect dramatically the quality of health care Americans receive by encouraging plans to compete on the basis of quality. At a time when new measures of quality may soon become available to patients, it is critically important that we examine how these measures may affect patients' choices and access to care.

Outcome Measures: Crucial but Can't Stand Alone

Some of the first measures available to consumers have been outcome measures. Examples of outcome measures include mortality rates from cardiac surgery, now publicly available in New York, and Cesarean section rates, now provided by many hospitals seeking to attract obstetric patients.

While making such measures available is critically important, making only outcome measures available would be woefully inadequate.

Using outcome measures alone creates strong incentives for health plans and health care providers to avoid sicker patients. Furthermore, they are not always a reliable measure of hospital or physician performance (Brook, McGlynn, & Cleary, 1996; Iezzoni, 1997). While Cesarean section rates depend on the ability of providers to deliver babies vaginally when the infant presents in a breech position, or when the mother has had a previous Cesarean section, the rates also depend on whether the hospital primarily serves low-risk pregnancies, high-risk pregnancies, or a mix of the two. Similarly, when surgeons are ranked by how frequently their patients die, it provides them with an incentive to take good care of their patients but it also provides them with an incentive to care only for well patients. Patients who have multiple health problems, who are older, or who are frailer are more likely to die during surgery than patients who are young and otherwise well. Past research already has shown that some health care plans do not provide the care needed by those with chronic conditions and that many markedly limit services (Fox, Wickes, & Newacheck, 1993a, 1993b; Horwitz & Stein, 1990).

Though the cardiac registry in New York has done an important job in risk-adjusting outcomes to help minimize the incentive for surgeons to turn away sicker and needier patients, risk adjusters are not available for all of the conditions on which outcomes are being measured or proposed. Outcome measures, when used alone, can have detrimental effects on the access of higher-risk and higher-need patients to care. They also can impact on patient choice. An example of this is the measure of how well a plan controls hypertension in the patients it serves. A 50-year-old, with marked hypertension, whose father died of a hemorraghic stroke, may be eager to begin medication, dietary changes and exercise to reduce his high blood pressure. An 89-year-old with asymptomatic high blood pressure and metastatic cancer may have little interest in or reason to change her diet to reduce blood pressure. Yet, the provider or plan whose quality is measured solely by outcome measures such as reduction in blood pressure, could face real pressures to urge the 89-year-old patient to take medications whose side effects outweigh the benefits, or to make dietary changes whose loss in quality of life make them not worth their gain in the patient's eyes. In sum, used in conjunction with other measures, a measure indicating that a plan reduces the blood pressure in a large number of its patients may be one good indicator of preventive care in that area. Used alone, an indicator counting the number of patients whose high blood pressure is controlled can provide incentives to limit patient choices.

What can be done? First, functional as well as clinical, outcome measures should be used (Nelson, Mohr, Batalden, & Plume, 1996) in a range of domains including cognitive, physical, social, and emotional (Newacheck et al., 1996). Understanding the impact of health care on patients' physical functioning, mental health, and their ability to care for themselves and their families, go to school, go to work, or be active in their communities is critical to understanding the impact on patients. Clinical outcome measures are most useful when they are strong predictors of long-term functional outcomes, new morbidity, or mortality.

Second, clinical outcome measures that are not skewed by differences in individual physiology, should be chosen. Laboratory results are often chosen for their convenience as outcome measures, but they often do not parallel the health outcome of concern. For example, even if 100% of patients with epilepsy were found to be in the therapeutic range for a given anticonvulsive medication, not all of them would be receiving appropriate treatment. Some would be having more toxic side effects than were necessary to control their seizures. Others might have their seizures ineffectively controlled. Less than 100% would be receiving high-quality care if by high-quality care we meant preventing seizures with the least side effects or, more appropriately, if we meant minimizing the impact of epilepsy on their lives while taking into account both the impact of potential seizures and potential medication side effects.

Third, to the extent possible, we need to select outcome measures that don't encourage plans and providers to serve only healthier, low-risk, and less needy patients. At present, the best means available for doing this are to select outcomes for diseases and treatments for which medical research has provided the information necessary to risk-adjust. The risk adjustment can be done in one of two ways. In mortality measures, where the relative risk of death attributable to age and comorbidities is known, a single number indicating reduction in anticipated mortality could be used. For the larger number of diseases in which it is known that certain populations are at much higher risk of poor outcomes, but for which the extent of their risk is not quantified, outcome measures could be disaggregated. For example, mortality rates could be presented separately for older patients and younger patients. Cesarean section rates could be presented separately for women giving birth to twins and women giving birth to singletons or, as has been done, for women who had previous vaginal deliveries and women who had previous Cesarean section deliveries.

Fourth, we need to recognize that risk adjustment is not perfect for any condition. Because of this, outcome measures should always be accompanied by access measures. They also will need to be accompanied by higher reimbursement rates to those providing care to sicker patients; otherwise the incentive to discourage treating these patients will remain. Reinsurance is one of the ways in which health care plans can receive the funding necessary to ensure that they provide adequate coverage to those with chronic conditions (Schlesinger & Mechanic, 1993).

Fifth, the potential impact on patient choice should be considered, particularly when selecting clinical measures. The best way to ensure that patients' values are respected while outcome goals are chosen is to include process measures. The process measures should include information provided by patients on whether their values were adequately taken into consideration in developing diagnostic and treatment plans whether they were encouraged to actively participate in decisions about their own care, as well as whether they were ever pressured into diagnostic or therapeutic plans that they did not want. Process measures will be discussed in more detail in the next section.

Process Measures: Needed to Enable Patients to Make Decisions About Their Own Lives

Consumers should be provided with information on the ways in which, and the extent to which, plans inform patients and encourage them to participate in decisions about their own care. As documented above, the evidence from research is strong. Patients want more information about their health conditions. Providing that information and building partnerships with patients is critical to their health as well as satisfaction.

Time spent with patients also proved to be an important factor in patient satisfaction and the likelihood of legal action (Levinson, Rotor, Mullooly, Dull, & Frankel, 1997). One study compared the communication skills of 59 primary care doctors and 65 surgeons with and without malpractice claims against them, demonstrating that among primary care physicians, those who spent time educating their patients, used humor, and actively facilitated their patients' involvement were less likely to have been sued in the past. Sixty-five percent of patients who sued, 63% of physicians who had been sued, and 62% of physicians who had not been sued agreed that better patient-doctor communication would reduce malpractice claims (Shapiro et al., 1989).

Furthermore, medical ethics and law are clear that "patients have well-recognized rights to be informed of their health status and to share in decisions about their care" (Emanuel, 1996, p. 241). The best way for patients to be able to exercise these rights is to receive information regarding which providers and plans encourage patient education and facilitate participation.

A number of managed care plans are now considering supplementing their list of physicians from which patients can choose with a brief biography of each physician. In addition to standard facts about a physician's medical education and training, some plans also have proposed including brief personal statements by physicians. In this context, it would be simple to ask physicians to include a statement on the extent and ways in which they involve patients in decisions about their own care. Such statements—combined with provider and plan-based measures of patient education, patient-provider communication, and patient participation—would both help patients make informed decisions and, by providing incentives to plans and providers, encourage patient education and participation, and improve patient health and satisfaction.

As in the case of outcome measures, process measures of quality should be presented in disaggregated form. The studies noted earlier highlight the greater problems faced by women, minorities, low-income patients, and those in poor health. Measures may need to be examined separately by race, class, and gender. Measures of how well a plan serves patients who are in poor health should also be presented separately from measures of how well they serve patients who are in good health. The mathematics of the problem are straightforward. If ninety-five percent of patients served by a plan are healthy and if the plan gets an "A" for the processes by which it serves these healthy patients, a plan could get an overall "A" on patient communication and participation, even if it received an "F" for patients who were sick. Yet, consumers might be particularly interested in how they would be treated when they were sick and in greatest need of high-quality care. Because of this, and because of the research documenting differential treatment of patients, process measures need to be disaggregated.

Access: Quality Has Little Meaning if Only the Healthy Get Access

There are two types of access problems. One type is whether all people, including individuals who currently are uninsured, can have access to care; the second type is whether consumers who are in a plan do in fact have access to the services that they believed they had when they signed up. A report card can help with the latter problem. Consumers need to have information on the characteristics of health plans that will affect their access to primary care, specialty care, diagnostic tests, and treatment. Unless consumers receive detailed information and report cards about practical access, and unless consumers have the opportunity to choose among plans based on this information, plans are likely to be more concerned about overuse of services than underuse. Research has shown that capitated physician groups are significantly more likely to monitor overuse (Kerr et al., 1996). Plans bear the costs of overuse, but patients bear the heaviest costs of underuse.

Consumers should have information on the rules and incentives under which physicians and other health care providers in the plan practice. The use of financial incentives has been clearly shown to influence whether physicians limit care (Hillman & Kerstein, 1989).

If plans work to increase the number of patients seen per hour and decrease the time health care providers spend with patients, this will affect the time that any given consumer is likely to have with their health care provider. Past research has shown that patients care about the amount of time they have with providers. Information about what is likely to influence provider time, as well as information on actual time spent by providers in a plan with patients, should be made available to consumers as they make their decisions. If primary care doctors are required by a plan's rules, or encouraged as a part of their performance evaluation, to see six patients an hour, then patients should be provided with this information. If a nurse practitioner's or a pediatrician's salary or bonus pay depends— whether through rules, regulations, performance reviews, financial incentives, or other mechanisms—on the number of patients they see in an hour, then the public should have access to this information. Medical ethicists have made clear both the importance of limiting physician and institutional conflicts of interests and providing full disclosure on potential conflicts of interest (Emanuel, 1996).

Time spent with primary care providers is only one small piece of the access issue. Plans also should provide information on rules, regulations, review processes, and financial incentives that may influence how likely a primary care practitioner is to refer a patient to a specialist (Cartland & Yudkowski, 1992). If the plan keeps track of how many times each primary care provider refers patients to a specialist, and uses this information as part of its review as to whether to keep primary care providers within the plan, these facts need to be known by patients. Similarly, if referral to specialists is limited or involves financial disincentives to the primary care physician or nurse practitioner, consumers deserve to know this. Information on the number and availability of specialists should be available. In the past, some plans have been criticized for hiring too few oncologists or other medical specialists who treat particularly sick patients in order to discourage those sick and costly patients from signing up for the plan. It is possible to contain costs without unnecessarily limiting visits to specialists, and without using primary care physicians as "gatekeepers," through such mechanisms as budgeting specialists into health care plans and educating patients about specialty visits (Bodenheimer, Lo, & Casalino, 1998).

Access to primary care providers and specialists are just two examples of ways in which plans may limit access to health care or expand access. Equally important are the incentives—whether through salary changes or through implications for job retention and promotion—and the rules and procedures which influence whether physicians recommend diagnostic tests or particular treatment options. Information on actual access to diagnostic and treatment opportunities should be provided, as well as information on incentives and procedures which may influence that access. Only through also examining measures such as waiting time for care, unjustified coverage denials, and waiting time for decisions regarding coverage will it be possible to examine the extent to which a plan limits the access to health care through indirect means (Grumet, 1989).

It is crucial that the services which are monitored for access encompass the services needed by those with chronic health conditions, and not just the services needed by those who are well. Past research has shown that capitated physician groups are more likely to monitor underuse of preventive services for those who are well than follow-up services for those with chronic conditions, even though follow-up services for those with chronic conditions play an equally important role in preventing further health problems (Kerr et al., 1996).

Information Needs to Be Comprehensible as Well as Comprehensive

The comprehensibility of the information is as essential as its comprehensiveness. Many factors go into making materials understandable. Once the material is written in understandable language, there are a number of different ways that the quantity of detailed information that consumers need can be provided.

User-friendly computer systems can now provide information readily to most people who can read. Computer technology is particularly well suited to allowing individuals to get the detailed information they want on specific health conditions or for specific patient populations, while not forcing them to go through a great deal of information that does not interest them. Programs can be designed so that a consumer who wants to know how well a plan treats young women of color can get that information, while another consumer can get information from the same program on how well a plan succeeds at treating patients with breast cancer.

Clearly, the same information can be provided in print format for those who do not want to or are unable to use computer technology. The principal disadvantage of the print format is that it does not readily allow the same tailoring to individual interests and questions.

Print and computers both require that the consumer be able to read and understand basic charts to be used independently. It is important that purchasers—Medicaid, Medicare, and employers—have individuals available to help get appropriate information to consumers who need to make a choice but can not read.

Patient Information: An Essential First Step, Not the Last Step Needed

Done correctly, providing high-quality information could make a critical difference in the ability of patients—both those with chronic conditions and those without—to choose plans and providers which will meet their health care needs. At the same time, it could enhance the ability of plans and providers to provide high-quality care. At present, with little information available to patients about quality, plans are forced to compete almost solely on the basis of cost. Those plans which want to provide more complete services or higher-quality care have the deck stacked against them if that care costs more money. Making a complete set of outcome, process, and access measures on all plans available to patients would mean that health care plans could compete on the basis of high quality as well as cost.

Yet, at the same time that we acknowledge the importance of providing patients and consumers with better information about health care plans and providers, we need to recognize that there are serious problems in the quality of care available to patients that will not be addressed by this free-market approach of competing on the basis of quality and cost. The most serious among these is access to affordable, high-quality care by those who have costly, chronic health conditions. The financial incentives, even with extensive public information on plans, will remain the same with regard to the care plans provided for those with the most costly chronic illnesses. Plans will continue to make more money if they are able to provide care principally to the healthy and to those with inexpensive chronic conditions. Even if the information available on their outcomes, processes, and access demonstrate that they do not provide good care to the minority of people who have serious, costly, chronic conditions, the majority of healthy consumers may still select them if they provide good care to those who are healthy. In fact, those who provide good care to patients with costly illness are likely to incur higher costs by attracting more such patients. This already has been seen in the past, and has ended in costly spirals for some of the insurers who have provided the best coverage to those with the worst conditions (Batavia, 1990). In testimony presented before the United States Senate during the health reform debates, it was noted that a Blue Cross plan whose actuarial value was $2,201 cost $3,720 because of adverse selection. As a result, those plans which provide better care to those with chronic conditions end up costing far more than plans which provide identical benefits, but serve a healthier patient population.

Report cards can improve quality of care for some patients, but they only will improve quality of care for all patients if they are combined with steps to ensure access for all. Quality measures always will provide information on the care received by the majority of patients, but they only will provide information on the quality of care experienced by all patients if measures of quality are disaggregated by gender, race, ethnicity, income, and health status. Disaggregating data is a critical first step; designing policies to ensure that plans and providers reach high quality standard for all patients—regardless of gender, race, ethnicity, income, or health status—is the crucial second step. The market alone will not protect subpopulations, particularly subpopulations that are as costly to treat as those with significant chronic conditions, diseases, or disabilities can be, or people who have no money with which to pay.

One of two approaches will be needed to address this problem. Either health care plans and insurance companies will need to receive enough additional money to cover those with chronic health conditions, so that they have an incentive to cover this population and can afford to do so while still competing for other patients (Luft & Miller, 1988) or regulations will be needed to limit the ability of insurers to exclude patients with costly chronic conditions from their plans. The Democratic and Republican bipartisan health insurance reform bill that passed was a first step in this direction. However, it was only a first step. While the bill required insurers to provide coverage to patients with chronic illness, plans could provide coverage at such a high cost that it would be unaffordable to most patients. Regulations such as community rating, or financial incentives such as those provided through risk adjustment and reinsurance, are necessary to ensure that patients with expensive chronic conditions have meaningful access to health care.

Finally, it is important to note that report cards can shed light on how one health plan measures up against another, but report cards alone will not help us answer an equally important question: how do health plans today and 10 years from now shape up against health plans 10 years ago. It is critically important that the American public receive report cards, not only on individual plans, but on our health care system. Patients need to receive information on how the quality of our health care system is changing over time (Brook, 1993) so that we as a country can evaluate whether the dramatic changes that are taking place in American health care are moving us forward, or only into a system where the sick get fewer services.

In the end, we should judge the success of report cards by assessing what impact they have on the experience patients have in a provider's office, examining room, or clinic; we should judge the report cards by how they affect the experience not of the majority of patients, but of all patients.

An Old Notion

Calling for developing partnerships with patients and investing time in those relationships is not new. Over two thousand years ago, Plato wrote in the *Laws*:

> Now have you observed that, as there are slaves as well as freemen among the patients of our communities, the slaves, to speak generally, are treated by slaves, who pay them a hurried visit, or receive them in dispensaries? A physician of this kind never gives a servant any account of his complaint, nor asks him for any; he gives him some empirical injunction with an air

of finished knowledge, in the brusque fashion of a dictator and then is off in hot haste to the next ailing servant—that is how he lightens his master's medical labors for him. The free practitioner . . . takes the patient and his family into his confidence. Thus he learns something from the sufferers, and at the same time, instructs the invalid to the best of his powers. He does not give his prescriptions until he has won the patient's support. (Hamilton & Cairns, 1961, pp. 1310–1311)

May we all treat our patients as free men, women, and children, and be treated that way when we become patients.

References

A committee of the environmental and occupational health assembly of the American Thoracic Society. (1996). Health effects of outdoor air pollution. *Amer J Resp Crit Care Med, 153,* 3–50.

Ad Hoc Committee on Health Literacy for the Council of Scientific Affairs, American Medical Association. (1999). Health Literacy: Report of the Council on Scientific Affairs. *JAMA, 281:6,* 552–557.

Administration on Aging. (1998). The Aging Network [online]. Available: www.aoa.dhhs.gov:80/aoa/webres/swsag.htm.

Ahmed, M., & Siegler, E. L. (1997). A revised bibliography for older individuals and their families. *Geriatrics, 52,* 43–50.

AIDS Institute, New York State Department of Health. (1995). *HIV and primary care: Putting prevention into practice.* Albany, NY.

American Association of Health Plans. *Number of people enrolled in HMOs, 1976–1996* [online]. Available: www.aahp.org/menus/index.cfm

American Association of Retired Persons. (1992). *A survey of the need for a prescription drug benefit under the Medicare program.* Washington, DC.

American College of Physicians-American Society of Internal Medicine. (1998). Making sense of Medicare and choice: HCFA's new managed care options confusing patients and doctors. *ACP-ASIM Observer, 1,* 12–13.

Andrew, M., Paes, B., & Johnston, M. (1990). Development of the hemostatic system in the neonate and young infant. *The American Journal of Pediatric Hematology/Oncology, 12*(1), 97.

Anonymous. (1998). HIV infections increasing among women and minorities. *HIV/AIDS Prevention.*

Anonymous. (1998). The HMO work group on case management. *Journal of the American Geriatrics Society, 46(3),* 303–308.

Anonymous. (1995). Disease Management cuts asthma inpatient rates. *Case Management Advisor 6(10),* 140–142.

Anonymous. (1994). Changes in U.S. demographics force cms to address patients' cultural diversity. *Case Management Advisor, 5*(11), 145–160.

Applegate, W. B., Blass, J. P., & Williams, T. F. (1990). Instruments for the functional assessment of older patients. *N Eng J Med, 322,* 1207–1214.

Baker, D. W., Parker, R. M., & Williams, M. V. (1996). The health care experience of patients with low literacy. *Archives of Family Medicine, 5,* 329–334.

Baker, D. W., Williams, M. V., Parker, R. M., Gazmararian, J. A., & Nurss, J. R. (in press). Development of a brief test to measure functional health literacy. *Patient Education and Counseling.*

Barnes, P. J., Pedersen, S., & Busse, W. W. (1998). Efficacy and safety of inhaled corticosteroids: New developments. *Amer J Resp Crit Care Med, 157,* S1–53.

Barnes, P. J. (1995). Inhaled glucocorticuids for asthma. *N Eng J Med, 302(86),* 868–875.

Barondess, J. A. (1993). The future of generalism. *Ann Intern Med, 119,* 153–160.

Barry, M. J., Mulley, A. G., Fowler, F. J., & Wennberg, J. W. (1988). Watchful waiting vw. immediate transurethral resection for symptomatic prostatism. *JAMA, 259(20),* 3010–3017.

Batavia, A. (1990). Health care reform and people with disabilities. *Health Affairs, 12,* 40–57.

Bauman, A. (1997). The comprehensibility of asthma education materials. *Patient Educ Couns, 32,* S51–S59.

Beasley, R., Cushley, M., & Holgate, S. T. (1989). A self-management plan in the treatment of adult asthma. *Thorax, 44,* 200–204.

Becker, M. H., & Maiman, L. A. (1975). Sociobehavioral determinants of compliance with health and medical care recommendations. *Medical Care, 1,* 10–24.

Benjamin, E. R. (1997). *Know Your rights in managed care: New York State's Consumers' Bill of Rights and utilization review.* New York, NY: The Legal Aid Society.

Berwick, D. M. (1996). Payment by Capitation and the Quality of Care. *N Eng J Med, 335,* 1227–1231.

Blumenthal, D. (1996). Quality of Care—What is it? *N Eng J Med, 335,* 891–894.

Blumenthal, D. (1996). The origins of the quality-of-care debate. *N Eng J Med, 335,* 1146–1149.

Blumenthal, D., & Epstein, A. M. (1996). The role of physicians in the future of quality management. *N Eng J Med, 335,* 1328–1331.

Bodenheimer, T. (1999). Disease management—Promises and pitfalls. *N Eng J Med, 340,* 1202–1205.

Bodenheimer, T., Lo, B., & Casalino, L. *Primary care physicians should be coordinators, not gatekeepers.* JAMA1999;281:2045–2049

Bozzette, S. A., Berry, S. H., Duan, N., Frankel, M. R,. Leibowitz, A. A., Lefkowitz, D., Emmons, C. A., Senterfitt, J. W., Berk, M. L., Morton, S. C., & Shapiro, M. F. (1998). The care of HIV-infected adults in the United States. HIV cost and services utilization study consortium. *N Eng J Med, 339(26),* 1897–1904.

Bradbury, E., Kay, S., Tighe, C., & Hewison, J. (1994). Decision making by parents and children in pediatric hand surgery. *British Journal of Plastic Surgery, 47,* 324–330.

Branch, L. G., Coulam, R. F., & Zimmerman, Y. A. (1995). The PACE evaluation: Initial findings. *The Gerontologist, 35,* 349–359.

Bringewatt, R. J. (1995). You have not yet begun to integrate. *Health Systems Review, 28(5),* 50–54.

Brod, M., & Heurtin-Roberts, S. (1992). Cross-cultural medicine: older Russian émigrés and medical care. *Western Journal of Medicine, 157,* 333–336.

Brody, D. S. (1980). The patient's role in clinical decision-making. *Ann Intern Med, 93,* 718–722.

Brody, D. S., Mille, S. M., Herman C. C., Smith, D. G., & Caputo, C. G. (1989). Patient perception of involvement in medical care. *Journal of General Internal Medicine, 4(6),* 506–511.

Brook, R., McGlynn, E., & Cleary, P. (1996). Measuring quality of care. *N Eng J Med, 335,* 966–970.

Brook, R. (1993). Maintaining hospital quality: The need for international cooperation. *JAMA, 270,* 985–987.

Butler, R. (1996). Foundations: A comprehensive approach to hemophilia care. Atlanta: Macro International.

Butler, C., Rollnick, S., & Stott, N. (1996). The practitioner, the patient, and resistance to change: recent ideas on compliance. *Canadian Medical Association Journal, 154,* 1357–1362.

Bycock, I. (1996). The nature of suffering and the nature of opportunity at the end of life. *Clinics in Geriatric Medicine, 12,* 237–252.

Calkins, D., Davis, R., & Reiley, P. (1997). Patient-physician communication at hospital discharge and patients' understanding of the postdischarge treatment plan. *Archives of Internal Medicine, 157,* 1026–1030.

Calkins, D. R., Rubenstien, L. V., Cleary, P. D., Davies, A. R., Jette, A. M., & Fink, A. (1991). Failure of physicians to recognize functional disability in ambulatory patients. *Ann Intern Med, 114,* 451–454.

Capozzi, J. M. (1997). Excerpts from: If you want the rainbow you gotta put up with the rain. JMC Industries Inc., p. 6. Distributed by American Airlines.

Carey, M. A., & Smith, M. W. (1992). Enhancement of validity through qualitative approaches: Incorporating the patient's perspective. *Evaluation and the Health Professions, 15,* 107–114.

Carey, R. M., & Engelhard, C. L. (1996). Academic medicine meets managed care: A high-impact collision. *Academic Medicine, 71(8),* 839–845.

Cartland, J., & Yudkowski, B. (1992). Barriers to pediatric referral in managed care systems. *Pediatrics, 89,* 183–192.

Caspar, G., & Brennan, P. (1994). Improving the quality of patient care: The role of patient preferences in the clinical record. *American Medical Informatics Association Proceedings,* 8–11.

Cassileth, B. R., Zupdis, R. V., Sutton-Smith, K., & March, V. (1980). Information and participation preferences among cancer patients. *Ann Intern Med, 92,* 832–836.

Centers for Disease Control and Prevention. (1998a). *The HIV/AIDS Epidemic in the United States, 1997–1998*. Rockville, MD: Author.

Centers for Disease Control and Prevention. (1998b). *HIV/AIDS Surveillance Report 10 (No.1) 10-19*. Rockville, MD: Author.

Chachkes, E., & Jennings, R. (1994). Latino communities; coping with death. In B. Dane & C. Levine (Eds.), *AIDS and the new orphans: Coping with death* (pp. 77–100). Westport, CT: The Greenwood Press.

Chassin, M. R. (1996). Part 3: Improving the quality of care. [Editorial]. *N Eng J Med, 335*(14), 1060–1063.

Cher, D. J., & Lenert, L. A. (1997). Method of Medicare reimbursement and the rate of potentially ineffective care of critically ill patients. *JAMA, 278*(12), 1001–1007.

Chow, J. (1999). Multiservice centers in Chinese-American immigrant communities: Practice principles and challenges. *Social Work, 44*(1), 70–80.

Christianson, J. B., Pietz, L., Taylor, R., Woolley, A., & Knutson, D. J. (1997). Implementing programs for chronic illness management: The case of hypertension services. *Joint Commission Journal on Quality Improvement, 23*(11), 593–601.

Clark, C. M., Jr., & Lee, D. A. (1995). Prevention and treatment of the complications of diabetes mellitus. *N Eng J Med, 332*, 1210–1217.

Clary, E. G., & Orenstein, L. (1991). The amount and effectiveness of help: The relationship of motives and abilities to helping behavior. *Person Soc Psychol Bulletin, 17*(1), 58–64.

Cleary, P. D., & Edgman-Levitan, S. (1997). Health care quality: Incorporating consumer perspectives. *JAMA, 278*(19), 1608–1614.

Cleary, P. D., Edgman-Levitan, S., Roberts, M., Moloney, T. W., McMullen, W., Walker, J. D., & Delbanco, T. L. (1991). Patients evaluate their hospital care: A national survey. *Health Affairs, 10*, 254–267.

Cleary, P. D., Greenfield, S., & McNeil, B. J. (1991). Assessing quality of life after surgery. *Controlled Clinical Trials, 12*, 189S–203S.

Cockrane, G. M. (1998). Compliance in asthma. *Eur Respir Rev, 8*, 239–242.

Cohen, E. L., & Cesta, T. G. (1997). *Nursing case management: From concept to evolution* (2nd ed.). St. Louis: Mosby-Year Book.

Cohen, K. (1997). *Integrated patient care concepts.* Paper presented at the Second Annual Washington Conference on Integrated Patient Care, Washington, DC, December 9–10.

Col, N., Fanale, J. E., & Hornhom, P. (1990). The role of medication non-compliance and adverse drug reactions in hospitalizations in the elderly. *Archives of Internal Medicine, 150*, 841–845.

Coons, S. J. (1996). Disease management: Definitions and exploration of issues. *Clinical Therapeutics, 18*(6), 1321–1326.

Counsel on Scientific Affairs for the American Medical Association. (1999). Health literacy: Report for the AMA council on scientific affairs. *JAMA, 281(6),* 552–557.

Crawford-Swent, C. (1996). Negotiating the chaos of patient care with clinical pathways. *Nursing Case Management, 1*(4), 173–179.

Cross, T. L., Bazron, B. J., Dennis, K. W., & Isaacs, M. R. (1989). Towards a culturally competent system of care. Washington, DC: CASSP Technical Assistance Center, Georgetown University Child Development Center.

Culbertson, R. A. (1996). How successfully can academic faculty practices compete in developing managed care markets? *Academic Medicine, 710*(8), 858–870.

Curtis, J. R., & Rubenfeld, G. D. (1997). Aggressive medical care at the end of life: Does capitated reimbursement encourage the right care for the wrong reason? *JAMA, 278*(12), 1025–1026.

Curtiss, F. R. (1997). Lessons learned from projects in disease management in ambulatory care. *American Journal of Health-System Pharmacists, 54,* 2217–2229.

Dallek, G. (1997). *The text of key state HMO consumer protection provisions: The best from the states.* Washington, DC: Families USA Foundation. http://www.familiesusa.org/best2.htm.

Davidoff, F.(1997). Time. *Ann Intern Med, 127,* 483–485.

Davidson, J. A. (1997). The treatment of type II diabetes in Texas: Current issues for managed care and employers. *Diabetes Care, 20*(3), 446–451.

Davis, T., Williams, M., Branch, W., & Green, K. (1999). Explaining illness to patients with limited literacy. In B. Whaley (Ed.), *Explaining illness: Research, theory, and strategies for comprehension.* Mahwah, NJ: Lawrence Erlbaum.

Davis, T. C., Long, S. W., & Jackson, R. H. (1993). Rapid Estimate of Adult Literacy in Medicine: A shortened screening instrument. *Family Medicine, 25,* 391–395.

Deber, R., Kraetschmer, N., & Irvine, J. (1996). What role do patients wish to play in treatment decision making? *Archives of Internal Medicine, 156,* 1414–1420.

Debusk, R. F., Miller, N. H., Superko, H. R., Dennis, C. A., Thomas, R.T., et al. (1994). A case-management system for coronary risk factor modification after acute myocardial infarction. *Ann Intern Med, 120*(9), 721–729.

Decastro, F. J. (1972). Doctor-patient communication: Exploring the effectiveness of care in a primary care clinic. *Clinical Pediatrics, 11,* 86–87.

Degner, L., Krisjanson, L., & Bowman, D. (1997). Information needs and decisional preferences in women with breast cancer. *JAMA, 277,* 1485–1492.

Deutsch, P., & Sawyer, H. (1990). *A guide to rehabilitation.* New York: Bender.

De Young, M. (1996) Research on the effects of pharmacist-patient communication in institutions and ambulatory care sites, 1969–1994. *American Journal of Health-System Pharmacists, 53,* 1277–1291.

Dilland, J. M. (1983). Multicultural counseling toward ethnic and cultural relevance in human encounters. (pp. 201–228). Chicago: Nelson-Hall.

Doak, C. C., Doak, L. G., & Root, J. H. (1996). *Teaching patients with low literacy skills* (2nd ed.). Philadelphia: Lippincott.

Donahue, D. C., Edelman, L. B., Ockene, I. S., & Saperia, G. (1996). Research collaboration between an HMO and an academic medical center: Lessons learned. *Academic Medicine, 71*(2), 126–132.

Dooha, S. J. (1998). *Managed care bill of rights for people with HIV.* New York: Gay Men's Health Crisis.

Eisenberg, D. M., Davis, R. B., Ettner, S. L., Appel, S., Wilkey, S., & Rompay, M. V. (1998). Trends in alternative medicine use in the United States, 1990–1997. *JAMA, 280*(18), 1569–1575.

Emanuel, L. (1996). A professional response to demands for accountability: Practical recommendations regarding ethical aspect of patient care. *Ann Intern Med, 124,* 240–249.

Eng, C., Pedulla, J., Eleazer, G. P., McCann, R., & Fox, N. (1997). Program of all-inclusive care for the elderly (PACER): An innovative model of integrated geriatric care and financing. *Journal of the American Geriatrics Society, 45,* 223–232.

Engel, G. L. (1977). The need for a new medical model: A challenge for biomedicine. *Science, 196,* 129–135.

Enslow, A. J., & Adler, L. M. (1972). Basic interviewing. In. A. Enslow & S. Swisher (Eds.), *Interviewing and patient care* (pp. 29–50). London: Oxford University Press.

Every, N. R. (1998). Influence of insurance type on the use of procedures, medications, and hospital outcome in patients with unstable angina: Results from the GUARANTEE registry. *Journal of the American College of Cardiology, 32,* 387–392.

Field, M. J., & Cassell, C. K. (1997). *Approaching death: Improving care at the end of life.* Washington, DC: National Academy Press.

Financing Task Force Retreat. (1998). The challenge of End-of-Life care: Moving Toward Metanoia? Washington, D.C.

Finkelmeier, B. A. (1995). *Cardiothoracic surgical nursing.* Philadelphia: J. B. Lippincott Company.

Finkler, K., & Correa, M. (1996). Factors influencing patient perceived recovery in Mexico. *Social Science and Medicine, 42,* 199–207.

Fontanarosa, P. B., & Lundberg, G. D. (1998). Alternative medicine meets science. *JAMA, 280*(18), 1618–1619.

Fox, H., Wick, L., & Newacheck, P. (1993a). Health maintenance organizations and children with special needs: A suitable match? *American Journal of Diseases of Children, 147,* 546–552.

Fox, H., Wicks, L., & Newacheck, P. (1993b). State Medicaid health maintenance organization policies and special needs children. *Health Care Financing Review, 15*, 25–37.

Freudenheim, M. (1998, April 24). Health insurers seek big increases in their premiums. New York Times.

Fries, J. F., Koop, C. E., Sokolov, J., Beadle, C. E., & Wright, D. (1998). Beyond health promotion: Reducing need and demand for medical care health care reforms to improve health while reducing costs. *Health Affairs, 17*(2), 70–84.

Gallant, J. E. (1999). The seropositive patient: The initial encounter. *HIV Clinical Management, 1* [On line]. Available: http://www.medscape.com.

Gazmararian, J., Baker, D., Williams, M., Parker, R. M., & Scott, T. L. (1999). Health literacy among Medicare enrollees in a managed care organization. *JAMA, 281*(6), 545–551.

Ginzberg, E., & Ostow, M. (1997). Managed care: A look back and a look ahead. *N Eng J Med, 336*, 1018–1020.

Givahn, R. D. (1992). The "reverend" of rap radio. *San Francisco Chronicle.*

Glasgow, R. E. (1995). A practical model of diabetes management and education. *Diabetes Care, 18*(1), 117–126.

Glassman, K., Shain, L., Carty, B., Ingram, D., Primack, S., Lloyd, M., Chachkes, E., & Gamble, M. (1998). *A continuum of care model for patients with heart failure (Final Report).* New York: United Hospital Fund.

Godoy, N., Howard, C., Cassino, C., Ciotoli, C., Ziegler, P., & Reibman, J. (1998). Asthma education in the emergency department improves patient knowledge and behavior. *Amer J Resp Crit Care Med, 157*, A837.

Goldzweig, C. L., Mittman, B. S., Carter, G. M., Donyo, T., Brook, R. H., Lee, P., & Mangione, C. M. (1997). Variations in cataract extraction rates in Medicare prepaid and fee-for-service settings. *JAMA, 277*(22), 1765–1768.

Gondolf, E. W. (1987). Evaluating programs for men who batter: Problems and prospects. *Journal of Family Violence, 2*, 95–108.

Gould, J. M., & Lomax, A. R. (1993). The evolution of peer education: Where do we go from here? *Journal of the American College of Health, 41*(6), 235–240.

Grahl, C. (1994). Improving compliance: Solving a $100 billion problem. *Managed Healthcare, 4*(6) (supplement), S11–S13.

Green, L. W. (1992). Prevention and health education. In Last, J. M., Wallace, R. B., et al. (Eds.), *Public health and preventive medicine* 13th ed. Norwalk, CT: Appleton and Lange, pp. 787–802.

Greene, M. G., Adelman, R. D., Friedmann, E., & Charon, R. (1994). Older patient satisfaction with communication during an initial medical encounter. *Social Science and Medicine, 38*(9), 1279–1288.

Greenfield, S., Kaplan, S., Ware, J., Yano, E., & Frank, H. (1989). In N. Goldfield & D. Nash (Eds.), *Providing quality care* (p. 448). Philadelphia: American College of Physicians.

Grumet, G. (1989). Health care rationing through inconvenience: The third party's secret weapon. *N Eng J Med, 321*, 607–611.

Guidry, G. G., Brown, W. D., Stogner, S. W., & George, R. B. (1992). Incorrect use of metered dose inhalers by medical personnel. *Chest, 101*, 31–33.

Gustafson, D., Hawkins, R., Boberg, E., Bricker, E., Pingree, S., & Chan, C. L. (1994). The use and impact of a computer-based support system for people living with AIDS and HIV infection. JAMA symposium supplement SCAMC proceedings. Philadelphia: Hanley and Belfus.

Gustafson, D., Wise, M., McTavish, F., Taylor, J. O., Wolberg, W., et al. (1993). Development and pilot evaluation of a computer-based support system for women with breast cancer. *Journal of Psychosocial Oncology, 11*, 69–93.

Hadley, E. C., Ory, M. G., Suzman, R., & Weindruch, R. (1989). Foreword. In E. C. Hadley, M. G. Ory, R. Weindruch, & L. Fried (Eds.), Symposium on physical frailty. *Journals of Gerontology, 48*, pp. (SI), vii-viii).

Hamilton, E., & Cairns, H. (1961). *Plato: The collected dialogues.* Princeton, NJ: Princeton University Press.

Harris, M. I. (1996). Medical care for patients with diabetes. *Ann Intern Med, 124*(1 Pt 2), 117–122.

Health Care Financing Administration. (1998). www.hcfa.gov/stats/hstats96/blustats.htm#trend.

Heymann, J. (1995). *Equal partners.* Boston: Little Brown and Company.

Hicks, L. L. (1993). *Role of the nurse in managed care.* Washington, DC: American Nurses Association.

Hillman, A., & Kerstein, J. (1989). How do financial incentives affect physicians' clinical decisions and the financial performance of HMOs? *N Eng J Med, 321*, 86–92.

HMO Workgroup on Care Management. (1998). Essential components of geriatric care provided through HMOs. *Journal of the American Geriatrics Society, 46*, 303–308.

Hoots, K. (1995). von Willebrand disease: An introduction. In Diagnosis and Management of Severe von Willebrand Disease. Symposium Proceedings. The National Hemophilia Foundation Annual Meeting, October 13, 1995, Philadelphia, PA.

Hoover, G. E., & Platts-Mills, T. A. E. (1995). What the pulmonologist needs to know about allergy. In R. J. Martin (Ed.), *Clinics in Chest Medicine.* Philadelphia: W. B. Saunders Company, pp. 603–620.

Hopper, S. (1993). The influence of ethnicity on the health of older women. *Clinics in Geriatric Medicine, 9*(1) 231–259.

Horn, S. D. (1996). Intended and unintended consequences of HMO cost-containment strategies: Results from the Managed Care Outcomes Project. *American Journal of Managed Care, 2*(3), 253–264.

Horwitz, S., & Stein, R. (1990). Health maintenance organization versus indemnity insurance for children with chronic illness. *American Journal of Diseases of Children, 144*, 581–586.

Houston-Miller, N. (1997). Strategies to enhance risk factor management in clinical practice. *The American Journal of Managed Care, 3*(sup), S70–S73.

Houston-Miller, N., Hill, M., Kottke, T., & Ockene, I. S. (1997). The multilevel compliance challenge: Recommendations for a call to action. *Circulation, 95*, 1085–1090.

Houts, P. S., Bucher, J. A., Mount, B., Britton, S., & Harvey, H. (1997). The Home Care Guide for Advanced Cancer. www.acponline.org.

HRSA Care ACTION. (1998). *Substance abuse and the HIV epidemic.* Washington, DC: Author.

Iezzoni, L. (1997). The risks of risk adjustment. *JAMA, 278*, 1600–1607.

Iglehart, J. K. (1995). Health policy report: Rapid changes for academic medical centers. *N Eng J Med, 332*(6), 407–411.

Iglehart, J. K. (1999) The American health care system. *N Eng J Med, 340*(5), 403–408.

Immunization Task Force. (1998). *Immunization management for managed care in the 21st century* (American Association of Health Plans White Paper).

Irish, D., Lundquist, K., & Nelsen, V. (1993). *Ethnic variations in dying, death and grief.* Washington, DC: Taylor and Francis.

Jette, A. M., Davies, A. R., Cleary, P. D., Calkins, D. R., Rubenstien, L. V., & Fink, A. (1986). The functional status questionnaire. *Journal of General Internal Medicine, 1*, 143–149.

Johnson, T. (1998). Shattuck Lecture: Medicine and the media. *N Eng J Med, 339*(7), 87–92.

Joint Commission for the Accreditation of Hospitals. (1993). *Accreditation manual for hospitals (Vol. I).* Oakbrook Terrace, IL: Author.

Joint National Committee on Prevention, Detection, Evaluation, and Treatment of High Blood Pressure, Sixth Report, National Heart, Lung and Blood Institute, National High Blood Pressure Education Program, NIH Publication #98-4080, November (1997).

Jones, J. G. (1983). Compliance with pediatric therapy: A selective review and recommendations. *Clinical Pediatrics, 22*, 262–265.

Joos, S., Hickam, D., Gordon, G., & Baker, L. (1996). Effects of a physician communication intervention on patient care outcomes. *Journal of General Internal Medicine, 11*, 147–155.

Kane, R. A., & Baker, M. O. (1996). *Managed care issues and themes: What next for the aging network? Highlights from the AOA-sponsored conference: Emerging Trends in Managed Care: Opportunities for the Aging Network* [Online]. Available: http://www.aoa.dhhs.gov/aoa/pages/mc-rpt.htm.

Kane, R. L., Kane, R. A., Finch, M., Harrington, C., Newcomer, R., Miller, N., & Hulbert, M. (1997). S/HMOs, the second generation: Building on the experience of the first social health maintenance organization demonstrations. *Journal of the American Geriatrics Society, 45,* 101–107.

Kaplan, S., Greenfield, S., Gandek, B., Rogers, W., & Ware, J. (1996). Characteristics of physicians with participatory decision-making styles. *Ann Intern Med, 124,* 497–504.

Kaplan, S., Greenfield, S., & Ware, J. J. (1989). Impact of the doctor-patient relationship on the outcomes of chronic disease. In M. Stewart & D. Roter (Eds.), *Communicating with medical patients.* Newbury Park, CA: Sage.

Kaplan, S. H., & Ware Jr., J. E. (1989). The patient's role in health care and quality assessment. In N. Goldfield & D. B. Nash (Eds.), *Providing quality care* (pp. 27–68). Philadelphia: American College of Physicians.

Kasper, J., Mulley, A., & Wennberg, J. (1992). Developing shared decision-making programs to improve the quality of health care, *Quality Review Bulletin, 18,* 183.

Kasteler, J., Kane, R. L., & Olsen, D. M. (1976). Issues underlying prevalence of "doctor-shopping" behavior. *Journal of Health and Social Behavior, 17,* 328–339.

Kavanagh, K., & Kennedy, P. (1992). Promoting cultural diversity. Newbury Park, CA: Sage.

Kerr, E. A., Mittmann, B. S., Hays, R. D., Leake, B., & Brook, R. H. (1996). Quality assurance in capitated physician groups: Where is the emphasis? *JAMA, 276,* 1236–1239.

Kilborn, P. T. (1998). Reality of H.M.O. system does not live up to hopes for health care. *New York Times.*

Kirsch, I., Jungeblut, A., Jenkins, L., & Kolstad, A. (1993). *Adult literacy in America: a first look at the results of the national adult literacy survey.* Washington, DC: National Center for Education Statistics.

Kitahata, M. M., Koepsell, T. D., Deyo, R. A., Maxwell, C. L., Dodge, W. T., & Wagner, E. H. (1996). Physicians' experience with the acquired immunodeficiency syndrome as a factor in patients' survival. *N Eng J Med, 334*(11), 701–706.

Kjellstrand, C. M., Kovithavongs, C., & Szabo, E. (1998). On the success, cost and efficiency of modern medicine: An international comparison. *Journal of Internal Medicine, 243,* 3–14.

Kleinman, A., Eisenberg, L., & Good, B. (1978). Culture, illness and care: Clinical lessons from cross cultural research. *Ann Intern Med, 88*(2), 251–258.

Kohler, C. L., Davies, S. L., & Bailey, W. C. (1995). How to implement an asthma education program. In R. J. Martin (Ed.), *Clinics in Chest Medicine.* Philadelphia: W. B. Saunders Co., pp. 557–565.

Kravitz, R., Hays, R., Sherbourne, C., DiMatteo, M. R., Rogers, W. H., Ordway, L., & Greenfield, S. (1993). Recall of recommendations and adherence to advice among patients with chronic medical conditions. *Archives of Internal Medicine, 153*(16), 1869–1878.

Kuczewski, M. G. (1998). Managed care and end-of-life decisions: Learning to live unplugged. *Archives of Internal Medicine, 158*, 2424–2428.

Kuttner, R. (1998). Must good HMOs go bad? *N Eng J Med, 338*, 1558–1563, 1635–1639.

Lachs, M. S., Feinstein, A. R., Cooney, L. M., Drickamer, M. A., Marottoli, R. A., & Pannill, F. C. (1990). A simple procedure for general screening for functional disability in elderly patients. *Ann Intern Med, 112*, 699–706.

Laine, C., Davidoff, F., & Lewis, E. A. (1996). Important elements of outpatient care: A comparison of patients' and physicians' opinions. *Ann Intern Med, 125*, 640–645.

Lamb, G. C., Green, S. S., & Heron, J. (1994). Can physicians warn patients of potential side effects without fear of causing those side effects? *Archives Internal Medicine, 154*, 2753–2756.

Landon, B. E., Wilson, I. B., & Cleary, P. D. (1998). A conceptual model of the effects of health care organizations on the quality of medical care. *JAMA, 279*(17), 1377–1382.

Landon, B. E., Tobias, C., & Epstein, A. M. (1998). Quality management by state Medicaid agencies converting to managed care: Plans and current practice. *JAMA, 279*(3), 211–216.

Lerman, C., Brody, D., Caputo, G., Smith, D., Lazaro, C., & Wolfson, H. (1990). Patient involvement in medical care. *Journal of General Internal Medicine, 5*, 29–33.

Levine, P., & Resnik, S., The Hemophilia Patient/Family Educational Model (PF Model). (1981). New York: The National Hemophilia Foundation. unpublished.

Levinson, W., Roter, D., Mullooly, J., Dull, V., & Frankel, R. (1997). Physician-patient communication: The relationship with malpractice claims among primary care physicians and surgeons. *JAMA, 277*, 553–559.

Lewis, C. C., Pantell, R. H., & Sharp, L. (1991). Increasing patient knowledge, satisfaction, and involvement: Randomized trial of a communication intervention. *Pediatrics, 88*, 351–358.

Lewis, S. J. (1984). Teaching patient groups. *Nursing Management 15*(5), 49–56.

Liaw, S., Young, D., & Farish, S. (1996). Improving patient-doctor concordance: An intervention study in general practice. *Family Practice, 13*, 427–431.

Lichter, S., & Lichter, L. (1988). *Television's impact on ethnic and racial images.* Washington, DC: American Jewish Committee.

Lindsey, B. J. (1997). Peer education: A viewpoint and critique. *Journal of the American College of Health, 45*(4), 1878–89.

Lipstak, G. S., & Revell, G. M. (1989). Community physician's role in case management of children with chronic illnesses. *Pediatrics, 84*, 465–471.

Longo, D. R., Land, G., Schramm, W., Fraas, J., Hoskins, B., & Howell, V. (1997). Consumer reports in health care: Do they make a difference in patient care? *JAMA, 278*(19), 1579–1584.

Lorig, K. (1996). *Chronic disease self-management: Case studies in applications for practice.* Picker Institute National Conference.

Luft, H., & Miller, R. (1988). Patient selection in a competitive health care system. *Health Affairs, 7,* 97–119.

Lush, M. T., Henry, S. B., Foote, K., & Jones, D. L. (1997). *Developing a generic health status measure for use in a computer-based outcomes infrastructure.* Paper presented at the 6th International Nursing Informatics Conference, Stockholm, Sweden.

Lusher, J., & Warrier, I. (1992). Hemophilia A. *Hematology/Oncology Clinics of North America, 6*(5), 1021–1033, 1022.

Lynch, M. A., & Ferri, R. S. (1997). Health needs of lesbian women and gay men—Providing quality care. *Clinician Reviews, 7*(1) [Online]. Available: www.medscape.com.

MacColl, W. A. (1996). *Group practice and prepayment of medical care.* Washington, DC: Public Affairs Press.

Mannino, D. M., Noma, D. M., Pertowski, C. A., Ashizawa, A., Nixon, L. L., Johnson, C. A., Ball, L. B., Jack, E., & Kang, D. S. (1998). Surveillance for Asthma—United States, 1960–1995. *Morbidity and Mortality World Reports, 47,* 1–27.

Manno, C. (1991). Difficult pediatric diagnoses: Bruising and bleeding. *Pediatric Clinics of North America, 38*(3).

Marinker, M. (1998). The current status of compliance. *Eur Respir Rev, 8,* 235–238.

Marlatt, G. A. (Ed.). (1998). *Harm reduction.* New York: Guilford.

Marquis, M., Davies, A. R., & Ware, J. E. Jr. (1983). Patient satisfaction and change in medical care provider: A longitudinal study. *Medical Care, 21,* 821–829.

Mathis, B. J. (1989). *Educational wants regarding family caregiving of women in Nebraska cooperative extension clubs.* Dissertation Abstracts International No. 50(04B) (University Microfilms International No. PUZ8918542).

Mayeaux, E. J., Jr., Murphy, P. W., Arnold, C., Davis, T. C., Jackson, R. H., & Sentell, T. (1996). Improving patient education for patients with low literacy skills. *American Family Physician, 53,* 205–211.

Mazur, D., & Hickam, D. (1997). Patients' preferences for risk disclosure and role in decision making for invasive medical procedures. *Journal of General Internal Medicine, 12,* 114–117.

McFadden, E. R. (1995). Improper techniques with metered dose inhalers: Clinical consequences and solutions to misuse. *J Allergy Clin Immunol, 96,* 277–283.

McHatton, M. (1985). A theory for timely teaching. *American Journal of Nursing, 20,* 798–800.

McLaughlin, L., & & Braun, K. (1998). Asian and Pacific Islander cultural values: Considerations for health care decision-making. *Health and Social Work, 23*(2), 116–126.

McNeill, P. (1993). *The ethics and politics of human experimentation.* New York: Cambridge University Press.

McTavish, F. M., Gustafson, D. H., Owens, B. H., Wise, M., Taylor, J. O., & Apantaku, F. M. (1994). Chess: An interactive computer system for women with breast cancer piloted with an under-served population. *American Medical Informatics Association Proceedings,* 599–603.

Miles, S. H., Weber, E. P., & Koepp, R. (1995). End-of-life treatment in managed care: The potential and the peril. *Western Journal of Medicine, 163,* 302–305.

Miller, C. (1991). *Inheritance of hemophilia.* New York: The National Hemophilia Foundation.

Mo, B. (1992). Modesty, sexuality and breast health in Chinese-American women. *Western Journal of Medicine, 157,* 323–327.

Montgomery R., Hilgartner, M. (1991). *Understanding vonWillebrand Disease.* New York: The National Hemophilia Foundation.

More, P. K., & Mandell, S. (1997). *Nursing case management: An evolving practice.* New York: McGraw-Hill Companies.

Moxley, D. P. (1994). Outpatient program development. In M. R. Donovan & T. A. Matson (Eds.), *Outpatient case management: Strategies for a new reality* (pp. 53–76). Chicago: American Hospital Publishing.

Mueller, C., Schur, C., & O'Connell, J. (1997). Prescription drug spending: The impact of age and chronic disease status. *American Journal of Public Health, 87,* 10, 16–26.

National Asthma Education and Prevention Program. (1997). Guidelines for the Diagnosis and Management of Asthma. Bethesda: National Institutes of Health, NHLBI.

National Hemophilia Foundation. (1998). *Participating in a clinical trial: Your life, your choice. A Guide for HIV Positive People.*

Nease, R., & Brooks, W. (1995). Patient desire for information and decision making in health care decisions. *Journal of General Internal Medicine, 10,* 593–600.

Nelson, E., Mohr, J., Batalden, P., & Plume, S. (1996). Improving health care: Part 1. The clinical value compass. *Journal on Quality Improvement, 22,* 243–258.

Nemeth, L., Hendricks, H., Salaway, T., & Garcia, C. (1998). Integrating the patient's perspective: Patient pathway development across the enterprise. *Topics in Health Information Management, 19*(2), 79–87.

Newacheck, P., Stein, R., Klein Walker, D., Gortmaker, S., Kuhlthau, K., & Perrin, J. (1996). Monitoring and evaluating managed care for children with chronic illnesses and disabilities. *Pediatrics, 98,* 952–958.

Nielsen Company. (1991). *Television viewing among blacks: The 1989–1990 television season.* Northbrook, IL: Author.

Ockene, I. S., Heebert, J. R., & Ockene, J. K. (1996). Effectiveness of physician training and a structured office practice setting on physician-delivered nutrition counseling: The Worcester-area trial for counseling in hyperlipidemia (WATCH). *American Journal of Preventive Medicine, 12*(4), 252–258.

O'Dowd, M. A. (1995). *AIDS mental health primer.* New York: Coalition of Voluntary Mental Health Agencies.

Ory, M. G., Schechtman, K. B., Miller, J. P., & Hadley, E. C. (1993). Frailty and injuries in later life: The FICSIT trials. *Journal of the American Geriatrics Society, 41*, 283–296.

Parikh, N. S., Parker, R. M., Nurss, J. R., Baker, D. W., & Williams, M. V. (1996). Shame and health literacy: The unspoken connection. *Patient Education and Counseling, 27*, 33–39.

Parker, R. M., Baker, D. W., Williams, M. V., & Nurss, J. R. (1995). The Test of Functional Health Literacy in Adults: A new instrument for measuring patients' literacy skills. *Journal of General Internal Medicine, 10*, 537–541.

Paterson, D. (1999). How much adherence is enough? A study of adherence to protease inhibitor therapy using MEMSCAPS. Paper presented at 6th Conference on Retroviruses and Opportunistic Infections. Chicago, February.

Petty, R., & Cacioppo, J. (1986). *Communication and persuasion: Central and peripheral routes to attitude change.* New York: Springer Verlag.

Phelan, G., Kramer, E. J., Grieco, A. J., & Glassman, K. S. (1996). Self-administration of medication by patients and family members during hospitalization. *Patient Education and Counseling, 27*, 103–112.

Pingree, S., Hawkins, R., & Gustafson, D. (1994). Will HIV-positive people use an interactive computer system for information and support? A study of CHESS in two communities. *American Medical Informatics Association Proceedings*, 22–26.

Prochaska, J. O., DiClimenti, C. C., & Norcross, J. C. (1992). In search of how people change: Applications to addictive behaviors. *American Psychologist, 57*, 1102–1114.

Public Law 102-73. (1991). *The National Literacy Act of 1991*, 102nd Congress, 1st Session.

Rand, C. S., Wise, R. A., & Nides, M. (1992). Metered dose inhaler adherence in a clinical trial. *American Review of Respiratory Diseases, 146*, 1559–1564.

Randall-Davis, E. (1989). *Strategies for working with culturally diverse communities and clients.* Office of Maternal and Child health.

Rawlings-Sekunda, J., Kaye, N., Riley, T., Scully, D., & Shed, S. (1997). *The lay of the land: What program managers need to know to serve people with HIV/AIDS in Medicaid managed care.* Portland, Maine: National Academy for State Health Policy.

Resnik, S. (1994). *The social history of hemophilia in the United States (1948–1988): The emergence and empowerment of a community.* Doctoral dissertation, Columbia University, New York.

Retchin, S. M., Brown, R. S., Yeh, S. J., Chu D., & Moreno, L. (1997). Outcomes of stroke patients under the Medicare fee for service and managed care. *JAMA, 278,* 119–124.

Rich, M. W., Beckham, V., & Wittenberg, C. (1995). A multidisciplinary intervention to prevent the readmission of elderly patients with congestive heart failure. *N Eng J Med, 333*(18), 1190–1195.

Riddick, S. (1999). Linguistic issues. In E. J. Kramer, S. L. Ivey, & Y. W. Ying (Eds.), *Immigrant women's health: Problems and solutions (pp. 35–43).* San Francisco, Jossey-Bass.

Rohling, M. L., & Binder, L. M. (1995). Money matters: A meta-analytic review of the association between financial compensation and the experience and treatment of chronic pain. *Health Psychology, 14,* 537–547.

Root, J. H. (1990) Developing low-literacy materials. In A. C. Matiella (Ed.), *Getting the word out: A practical guide to AIDS materials development* (pp. 63–77). Santa Cruz, CA: Network Publications.

Rosenstock, I. M., Strecher, V. J., & Becker, M. H. (1998). Social learning theory and the health belief model. *Health Education Quarterly, 15*(2), 175–183.

Rosenstreich, D. L., Mitchell, H., McNiff-Mortimer, K., Lynn, H., Ownby, D., Malveaux, F., Eggleston, P., Kattan, M., Baker, D., Slavin, R. G., Gergen, P., Mitchell, H., McNiff-Mortimer, K., Lynn, H., Ownby, D., & Malveaux, F. (1997). The role of cockroach allergy and exposure to cockroach allergen in causing morbidity among inner-city children with asthma. *N Eng J Med, 336,* 1356–1363.

Roter, D., Hall, J., Kern, D., Barker, L., Cole, K., & Roca, R. (1995). Improving physicians' interviewing skills and reducing patients' emotional distress. *Archives of Internal Medicine, 155,* 1877–1884.

Rousseau, P. (1998). Palliative care in managed Medicare: Reasons for hope and for concern. *Geriatrics, 53,* 59–65.

Rubin, R. J., Altman, W. M., & Mendelsohn, D. N. (1994). Health care expenditures for people with diabetes mellitus. *J Clin Endocrinol Metab, 78,* 809A–809F.

Ruckdeschel, J., Albrecht, T., Blanchard, C., & Hemmick, R. (1996). Communication, accrual to clinical trials, and the physician-patient relationship. *Journal of Cancer Education, 11,* 73–79.

Rush, A. G., & Cappello, D. (1990). Telling a tale. In A. C. Matiella (Ed.), *Getting the word out: A practical guide to AIDS materials development* (pp. 103–112). Santa Cruz, CA: Network Publications.

Satinsky, M. A. (1995). *An executive guide to case management strategies.* Chicago: American Hospital Publishing, Inc.

Sawyer, R. G., Pinciaro, P., & Dedwell, D. (1997). How peer education changed peer sexuality educator's self esteem, personal development, and sexual behavior. *Journal of the American College of Health, 45*(5), 211–217.

Schappert, S. M. (1997). Ambulatory care visits to physician offices, hospital outpatient departments, and emergency departments: United States, 1995. *Vital Health Statistics, 13*(129).

Schlesinger, M., & Mechanic, D. (1993). Challenges for managed competition from chronic illness. *Health Affairs, 12* Suppl, 123–137.

Schneider, E. C., & Epstein, A. M. (1996). Influence of cardiac surgery performance reports on referral practices and access to care: A survey of cardiovascular specialists. *N Eng J Med, 335*(4), 251–256.

Schultz, R. K. (1995). Drug delivery characteristics of metered-dose inhalers. *J Allergy Clin Immunol, 96*, 284–287.

Shapiro, R., Simpson, D., Lawrence, S., Talsky, A., Saboncinski, K., & Schneidermayer, D. (1989). A Survey of Sued and Nonsued Physicians and Suing Patients. Arch Intern Medicine, 149, 2190-2196.

Shaughnessy, P. W., Crisler, K. S., Schlenker, R. E., & Arnold, A. G. (1997). Outcomes across the care continuum: Home health care [see comments]. *Medical Care, 35*(11 Suppl), NS115–23.

Silliman, R., Troyan, S., Guadagnoli, E., & Kaplan, S. (1997). The impact of age, marital status, and physician-patient interactions on the care of older women with breast carcinoma. *Cancer, 80*, 1326–1334.

Simon, S. R., Pan, R. J., Sullivan, A. M., Clark-Chiarelli, N., Connelly, M. T., et al. (1999). A survey of students, residents, faculty and deans at medical schools in the United States. *N Eng J Med, 340*, 928–936.

Simons-Morton, B. G., Greene, Walter, H., & Gottlieb, N. H. (1995). *Introduction to health education and health promotion.* Prospect Heights: Waveland Press.

Sloane, B. C., & Zimmer, C. G. (1993). The power of peer health education. *Journal of the American College of Health, 41*(6), 241–245.

Soucie, J. M., Evatt, B., & Jackson, D. (1998). Occurrence of Hemophilia in the United States. *American Journal of Hematology, 59*, 288–294.

Sowell, R., & Meadows, T. (1994). An integrated case management model: Developing standards, evaluation and outcome criteria. *Nursing Administration Quarterly, 18*(2), 53–64.

Stanley, J. (1998). The American health decision, quest to die with dignity. Appleton, WI: publisher.

Stedman, L., & Cassel, C. (1991). Literacy and reading performance in the United States from 1880 to present. In C. Kaestle (Ed.), *Literacy in the United States: Readers and readings since 1880* (pp. 75–128). New Haven: Yale University Press.

Stewart, A., Greenfield, S., & Hays, R. (1989). Functional status and well-being of patients with chronic conditions: Results from medical outcomes study. *JAMA, 262*, 907–913.

Stoeckle, J. (1993). Improving communication with patients. *Forum, 14*, 7–8.

Street, R. L. (1992). Communicative styles and adaptations in physician-parent consultations. *Social Science and Medicine, 34*, 1155–1163.

Stuart, M. R., & Lieberman, J. R. (1993). *The fifteen-minute hour: Applied psychotherapy for the primary care physician* (2nd ed.). New York: Praeger.

Support Principal Investigators. (1995). A controlled trial to improve care for seriously ill hospital patients. *JAMA, 274*(20), 1591–1598.

Tarlov, A., Ware, J. J., Greenfield, S., Nelson, E., Perrin, E., & Zubkoff, M. (1989). The medical outcomes study: An application of methods for monitoring the results of medical care. *JAMA, 262*, 925–930.

The Boston Consulting Group. (1995). *The promise of disease management.* Boston, MA: The Boston Consulting Group Inc.

Teplitz, L., Egenes, K. J., & Brask, L. (1990). Life after sudden death: The development of a support group for automatic implantable cardioverter-defibrillator patients. *Journal of Cardiovascular Nursing, 4*(2), 20–32.

Thomas, T. (1997). *Cardiovascular risk reduction: A nurse-managed, physician-directed model.* Paper presented at the Second Annual Washington Conference on Integrated Patient Care, Washington, DC.

Tobin, D. R. (1999). *Peaceful dying: The step-by-step guide to preserving your dignity, your choice, and your inner peace at the end of life.* Reading, MA. Perseus Books.

Todd, W. E., & Nash, D. (Eds.). (1997). *Disease management: A systems approach to improving patient outcomes.* Chicago: American Hospital Publishing.

U.S. Bureau of the Census, 1993.

Vace, N. A., DeVaney, S. B., & Wittmar, J. (1995). *Experiencing and counseling multicultural and diverse populations* (3rd ed.). Bristol, PA: Accelerated Development.

Varner, K. S. (Ed.). *Curriculum Directory 1998–1999.* Washington, DC: American Association of Medical Colleges.

Ward, M. D., & Rieve, J. A. (1997). The role of case management. In W. E. Todd & D. Nash (Eds.), *Disease management: A systems approach to improving patient outcomes* (pp. 235–260). Chicago: American Hospital Publishing.

Webster, J. R., & Feinglass, J. (1997). Stroke patients, managed care, and distributive justice. *JAMA, 278*(2), 161–162.

Wechlsler, H., Levine, S., & Idelson, R. (1996). The physician's role in health promotion revisited: A survey of primary care practitioners. *N Eng J Med, 334*(15), 996–998.

Weed, R., & Riddick, S. (1992). Life care plans as a case management tool. *The Case Manager, 3*(1), 28–31.

Weeks, S. K. (1995). What are the educational needs of prospective family caregivers of newly disabled adults? *Rehabilitation Nursing, 20*(5), 256–260.

Weingarten, S. (1997). *Clinical guidelines.* Paper presented at the Second Annual Washington Conference on Integrated Patient Care, Washington, DC.

Weiss, B. D., & Coyne, C. (1995). *Experimental treatments for HIV and AIDS.* Albany, NY: AIDS Institute.

Weiss, B. D., & Coyne, C. (1997). Communicating with patients who cannot read. *N Eng J Med, 337,* 272–274.

Weiss, K. B., Gergen, P. J., & Hodgson, T. A. (1992). An economic evaluation of asthma in the United States. *N Eng J Med, 326,* 862–866.

Wennberg, J., & Gittelsohn, A. (1975). Health care delivery in Maine I: Patterns of Use of Common Surgical Procedures. *Journal of the Maine Medical Association, 56*(5), 123–149.

Wennberg, J., & Gittelsohn, A. (1973). Small area variations in health care delivery. *Science, 162,* 1102–1108.

Westberg, J., & Jason, H. (1996). Influencing health behavior: The process. In Woolf, S. H., Jonas, S., & Lawrence, R. S. (Eds.), *Health promotion and disease prevention in clinical practice.* Baltimore: Williams & Wilkins, 145–162.

Williams, M. V., Baker, D. W., Honig, E. G., Lee, T. M., & Nowlan, A. (1998). Inadequate literacy is a barrier to asthma knowledge and self care. *Chest, 114,* 1008–1015.

Williams, M. V., Baker, D. W., Parker, R. M., & Nurss, J. R. (1998). Relationship of functional health literacy to patients' knowledge of their chronic disease: A study of patients with hypertension or diabetes. *Archives of Internal Medicine, 158,* 166–172.

Williams, M. V., Parker, R. M., Baker, D. W., Pitkin, K., Coates, W. C., & Nurss, J. R. (1995). Inadequate functional health literacy among patients at two public hospitals. *JAMA, 274,* 1677–1682.

Wilson, S. R. (1998). Individual versus group education: Is one better? *Patient Education and Counseling, 32,* S67–S75.

Wittmar, J. (1995). Older order Amish: Culturally different by religion. In Vace, N., De Vaney, S., & Wittmar, J., (Eds.), *Experiencing and counseling multicultural and diverse populations.* Bristol, PA: Accelerated Development.

Woolf, S. H., Jonas, S., & Lawrence, R. S. (1996). *Health promotion and disease prevention in clinical practice.* Baltimore: Williams and Wilkins.

Zalta, E., Eichner, H., & Henry, M. (1994). New trends in disease management. Managing Employee Health Benefits, Winter.

Zander, K. (1995). Collaborative care: Two effective strategies for positive outcomes. In K. Zander (Ed.), *Managing outcomes through collaborative care* (pp. 1–38). Chicago: American Hospital Publishing, Inc.

Index

Page numbers followed by "t" indicate tables.

247